STANDOFF:
Virus and Us

STANDOFF:
Virus and Us

Editor: Bharat S. Thakkar, Ph.D.

To order additional copies of this book, contact:
Xlibris
844-714-8691
www.Xlibris.com
Orders@Xlibris.com
838230

Dedication

This book is dedicated to the business managers who helped this world a better place to live and work and to those in coming decades who would help make it better for the generations to come. Special thanks are due to its contributing authors named alphabetically below:

Akesh, Arvindbhai, Deepal, Indraine, Jayantbhai, Kadambari, Kevin, Kunj, Lydia, Mayankbhai, Nicolas, Toni, and their families. Without their dedication and cooperation, such work is impossible to create in these times of hardships and uncertainties.

Bharat S. Thakkar, Ph.D., Editor

Change is the law of life and those who look only to the past or present are certain to miss the future
—John F. Kennedy

Slowness to change usually means fear of the new.
—Philip Crosby

The key to change . . . is to let go of fear
—Rosanne Cash

If you don't like something, change it. If you can't change it, change your attitude
—Maya Angelou

CONTENTS

List of Figures xi

List of Tables...xii

Notes on Contributors...xiii

Foreword: by Kevin Sorbello xxxiii

Preface: by Bharat Thakkar...xxxix

Introduction: by Lydia Daniels..xlix

Chapter 1   COVID-19 Pandemic Complexity:
             The Tipping Point for Decision-Making
             By Kadambari Ram......................................1

Chapter 2   Business and Social Challenges
             from Unexpected Global Events
             By Kevin M. Sorbello...................................38

Chapter 3   Impact of COVID-19 on Global Gig Economy
             By A. C. Brahmbhatt 84

Chapter 4   Economic Impact of a Pandemic:
             Survival and Recovery
             By Toni McIntosh 121

Chapter 5   Impact of COVID-19 on Technology Startups
             and Technology Entrepreneurship in India
             By Deepal Joshi...144

Chapter 6   Change Management Complexities during
             Pandemic Faced by Managers and Leaders
             By Indranie Gurusamy Ram 193

Chapter 7   COVID-19: Clinician's Perspective
             and Impact on Healthcare Workers
             By Akesh Thomas and Jay Mehta.............................222
Chapter 8   Understanding the Effects of Coronavirus
             from a Virological and Public Health Perspective
             By Kunj R. Patel..248
Chapter 9   Quantum Computers—Using Change
             Management to Study the Pandemic
             By Nicolas M. Casati and Kevin M. Sorbello 273
Chapter 10   A Journalist's Perspective: COVID-19
             and How It Upended the World
             By Mayank Chhaya...305

Index..329

LIST OF FIGURES

Chapter 2

Figure 1. The Structure of the COVID-19 Virus............................40
Figure 2. Deaths per 1000 in the US 2019-2021............................52
Figure 3. Deaths per 1000 in the US 2013-2021 53
Figure 4. Deaths per 1000 in the US 2000-2021 53
Figure 5. Deaths per 1000 in the US 2000-2021 (0 – 10 scale)........54

Chapter 5

Figure 1. Fintech Entrepreneurship in India during COVID-19.... 152
Figure 2. Edtech Entrepreneurship in India during COVID-19 153
Figure 3. Healthtech Entrepreneurship in India during
         COVID-19.. 154
Figure 4. Online Retail Entrepreneurship in India during
         COVID-19.. 155
Figure 5. SaaS and Remote-Working Tools Entrepreneurship
         in India 155
Figure 6. OTT Platforms, Online Gaming and Vernacular
         Podcasting 156
Figure 7. Five Years Comparative Picture of Total Funding in
         Billion Dollars and Number of Funding Rounds for
         Technology Start-ups in India 157
Figure 8. Examples of Technology Start-ups Pivoting During
         COVID-19 in India 176
Figure 9. Four Levels of Resilience for Entrepreneurial
         Growth during Crisis 177

LIST OF TABLES

Chapter 5

Table 1. Immediate and Long-term Impacts of COVID-19 on
Technology and Information Technology Sectors 147

Table 2. Innovative Solutions by Technology Start-ups to
Combat COVID-19 in India 160

Table 3. Challenges and Survival Strategies of Technology
Startups during COVID-19 in India – Part 1 164

Table 4. Challenges and Survival Strategies of Technology
Startups during COVID-19 in India – Part 2 166

Table 5. Government of India Policy Measures for Technology
Start-ups during COVID-19 in India. Source: Start-up
India, 2021; Invest India, 2020 169

Table 6. Long-term Effects of Select Technologies Beyond
COVID-19: Technologies for Saving Life and
Improving Health 173

Table 7. Long-term Effects of Select Technologies Beyond
COVID-19: Technologies for Improving Quality of Life 174

Table 8. Role and Significance of Components of Technology
Entrepreneurship 179

Table 9. Studies from Several Nations on Technology Start-
ups & Technology Entrepreneurship during COVID-19 181

Chapter 8

Table 1. Advantages and Disadvantages
of Different Vaccine Platforms 260

NOTES ON CONTRIBUTORS

A. C. Brahmbhatt, Ph.D.

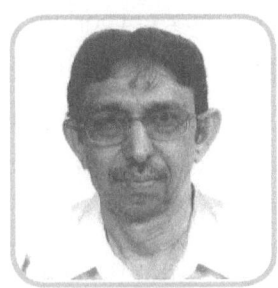

Dr. A. C. Brahmbhatt is in the field of academics for the last 5 decades, busy teaching the master's courses, publishing research papers, guiding Ph. D. students and acting as research mentor the universities located in Gandhinagar, India. He had his M.Sc. from Maharasja Sayajirao University of Baroda, India (1967), Ph.D. from Gujarat University (1981) and FDP for Indian Institute of Management, Ahmedabad (IIMA), 1982. He was Head of Marketing Area at BK School of Business Management (India), Chairman of Doctoral Program in Management of Nirma University, India (2009-16) and currently the Research Mentor of two universities, one being Pandit Dindayal Energy University (PDEU) and Kadi Sarv Visvavidyalaya both in Gandhinagar, India.

He had taught various programs like MBA, M.Phil., Ph.D. in leading management and entrepreneurship institutes like BK School, CEPT, National Institute of Fashion Design (NIFT), Mudra Institute of Communication, Ahmedabad (MICA), Entrepreneurship Development Institute of India (EDI-I) etc. He taught variety of courses such as Marketing Research and Information System (MRIS), Research

Methodology, Consumer Behavior, Services Marketing, Operations Research, Inventory Management etc. He has published 34 research papers in the leading management journals, India and abroad. He has produced 10 Ph.D.'s in the area of marketing so far. He is on 8 Boards of Editorial and Reviewer Boards, India and abroad. He has provided consultancy services to various corporate, governmental and non-governmental units such as Oil India Limited (OIL), ISRO, Gujarat State Civil Supply Corporation (GSCSC), Industrial Extension -Cottage (INDEXT-C), Self Employed Women Association (SEWA), Aims Oxygen Ltd. etc.

He has got Biographical Entry into, i) Reference Asia Who's Who of Men and Women of Achievement, Volume IV, (1992), ii) Reference India-Biographical Note on Men and Women of Achievement of Today and Tomorrow, Vol.1, Page. 129, iii) Indo Europe's Who's Who, 1995, iv) Learned India-Distinguished Biographies in Twenty First century, 2010.

He has been awarded the best paper awards in Applied Statistics consecutively for two years 1978 and 1979. Also, he has been awarded,' Best Professor of Marketing, Dainik Bhaskar National Educational Leadership Award, 'October13, 2013, Mumbai, India.

He as a Chairperson of Doctoral program at Nirma University had organized 6 annual Doctoral Conferences, called ANVESH. He is one of the founder promoters and trustees of Consumer Education and Research Centre (CERC) - a renowned consumer forum situated in Ahmedabad, India.

Nicolas Casati, DBA

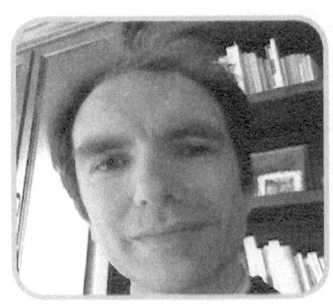

Nicolas M. Casati DBA, has 20 years of experience at a 30,000 employee Healthcare System in the Chicago area. Dr. Casati is a recognized expert in decontamination of surgical instruments, as a Certified Registered Central Service Technician and Certified Healthcare Leader by the International Association of Healthcare Central Service Material Management. Dr. Casati is consulted by surgical equipment manufacturers and has contributed two process improvements at the Healthcare System: environmental and staff related. In addition to experience working at an International Bank as an intern, volunteering as an Occupational Safety Training Presenter, and being certified CompTIA A+ 1001, Dr. Casati has three years of Information Systems experience and in 2021, trained on Arduino IDE and TinkerCAD, (the Internet of Things). Using his knowledge learned during his Environmental Sciences studies, Dr. Casati has advised on 200 manuscripts as a reviewer of the Journal of Cleaner Production and particularly interested in Corporate Social Responsibility. Dr. Casati is creative, with two patent filings in regard to noise control, assigned to Woxx Incorporated, a start-up company at which he is President. Dr. Casati is Vice-President at the Groupe Professionnel Francophone in Chicago. He has done volunteer work in a hospital in Honduras".

Mayank Chhaya, Renowned Journalist

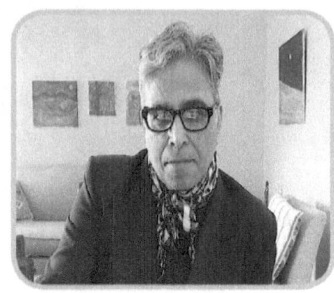

Mayank Chhaya is a respected journalist and writer with four decades of reporting out of India, Pakistan, Sri Lanka, and the United States. He has reported all major news stories out of India since 1982. He is a widely published commentator on global affairs but in particular on South Asian, Chinese and Sino-Tibetan affairs.

He is also an authorized biographer of the Dalai Lama whose book 'Man, Monk, Mystic' has been published in 24 languages around the world, including in America by Random House. The book has been updated with four new chapters under a new title 'The Dénouement: The 14th Dalai Lama's life of persistence' and is available at Amazon.

Chhaya is also the writer, director, editor and cameraman of a feature-length critically acclaimed documentary titled 'Gandhi's Song' which is now going through international distribution.

He is currently working on three more books. Chhaya also hosts a widely watched online news show 'Mayank Chhaya Reports'.

As a journalist, Chhaya has also extensively reported on the COVID pandemic from many different angles. In his chapter he brings to bear his long years in journalism to offer a broad view of how the pandemic has fundamentally affected our lives.

Lydia M. Daniels, Ph.D.

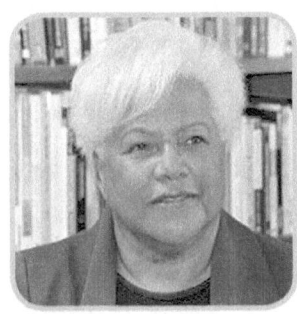

Dr. Lydia M. Daniels, Ph.D., is currently President and CEO, Daniels Consultation Services, Atwater, CA; Distinguished Adjunct Professor, Golden Gate University, San Francisco, CA, Ageno School of Business, Human Resources Management; and former Adjunct Professor, Dominican University of California, San Rafael, CA., Barowsky School of Business. Lydia provides consultation and project management services for a variety of organizations for over a twenty-five-year period. She has held top-level positions such as Chief Human Resources Officer for a 3000-employee healthcare system and demonstrated expertise in development and implementation of major HR systems, organizational transition projects, and union contract negotiations and implementation. She teaches graduate courses in Strategic Human Resource Management, Performance Management, and Organizational Behavior, in both cyber and classroom. She is experienced in course and curriculum development in Human Resource Management. She holds an MS in human resources management and Ph.D. in management/leadership and organization change. The recipient of the Management Fellowship Award from the University of California, San Francisco 1979-1980, Dr. Daniels was recognized as the Woman of the Year by the National Association of Professional Women in 2012, among the Outstanding Adjunct Faculty for the Human Resources Program by the Edward S. Ageno School of Business in 2016 and as a Distinguished Adjunct Professor by Golden Gate University in 2018 and was also presented with the 2020-2021 Albert Nelson Marquis Lifetime Achievement Award by Marquis Who's Who.

Additionally, she is scheduled as a presenter at the International Servant Leadership Summit, 2021. As a disciple of Servant Leadership, she has authored: The Quest for a Paradigm Shift in Leadership, (Chapter 3), in Bharat S. Thakkar, (Ed.), The Future of Leadership: Addressing Complex Global Issues, 2018, Palgrave / Macmillan, and author of 21st Century Global Human Resource Management: Strategic Business Partner and Servant Leader (Chapter 3) in Bharat S. Thakkar, (Ed.), Paradigm Shift in Management Philosophy: Future Challenges in Global Organizations, 2020, Palgrave / Macmillan Publisher. Dr. Daniels is incredibly proud of developing and delivering graduate courses for the Master of Science in Human Resource Management program at Golden Gate University and promoting the philosophy and practice of Servant Leadership in professions, organizations, communities, and the world.

Deepal Joshi, Ph.D.

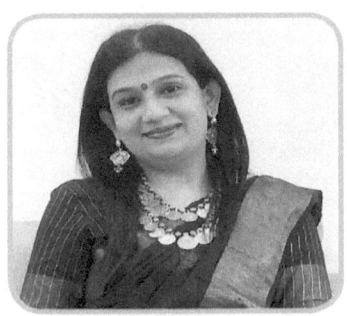

Dr. Deepal Joshi is a Management Faculty at Somlalit Institute of Business Administration, affiliated to the Gujarat University, situated in Ahmedabad, Gujarat State, India; where she also serves as the Director-in-Charge for Management under-graduate studies. Besides being a gold medalist at management under-graduate and graduate study, she has completed her doctorate on 'Trends in B2C e-Commerce'. She has more than two decades of teaching experience for management students at the undergraduate studies. She has also played diverse roles as examination coordinator and chairman of the syllabus revision committees for management courses.

Her research focuses on trends in B2C e-commerce, e-loyalty, website usage experiences of e-buyers, leadership in Indian high-tech start-ups, women entrepreneurs in Indian high-tech start-ups and governance of higher education in India. In addition to conference presentations, her publications and book chapters are associated with several reputed national and international journals. She can be reached by email at deepal2277@gmail.com

Toni McIntosh, Ph.D.

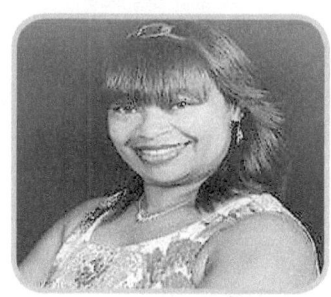

Dr. Toni McIntosh is a graduate of Shaw University in Raleigh, North Carolina, where she earned a Bachelor of Science degree in Business Management. She further matriculated to the University of North Alabama in Florence, Alabama, where she earned an MBA in International Business. In 2020, she earned a PhD in Management from Walden University in Minneapolis, Minnesota. Dr. McIntosh has worked for state agencies and private sector businesses in North Carolina in the Information Technology industry for 22 years, primarily in Security Administration and Access Management. She has spent the last 12 years working in IT in the healthcare industry as an Information Technology Analyst at UNC Health in North Carolina, a leading teaching hospital affiliated with the University of North Carolina at Chapel Hill. She is a leader in her church, and actively serves on several ministries there, and is the managing editor of the church newsletter, The Calvary Chronicle. Dr. McIntosh has a predilection for assisting and encouraging junior high and high school students in planning for their education and work success. She has a zeal for workplace equality with a special interest in cultural, gender, and age inequalities. A native of New Jersey, she now resides in North Carolina with her two parakeets.

Dr. Jayant Mehta, MD

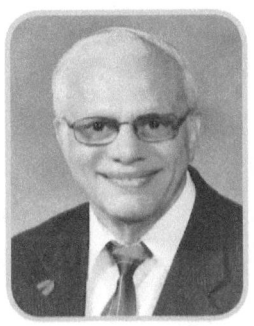

Dr. Jayant Mehta received his medical degree from MS university of Baroda, India. After spending a year as a medical officer in Jinja, Uganda, he came to USA in 1971. After three years of training in IM at SUNY, Stony Brook, NY, he went to Denver, Co for a research fellowship in Tuberculosis. He became a pulmonary specialist and a founding faculty member at the COM of the East Tennessee State University at Johnson City, TN. He had notable experience in communicable diseases like Malaria, Sleeping sickness and Tuberculosis in East Africa. His research training in Tuberculosis at the National Jewish hospital in Denver, Co. added to his experiences in TB.

After coming to Johnson City, TN, Dr. Mehta started TB treatment and prevention program in East TN and served as the medical director for 37 years. He is also a founding board member of the Tricities Temple in East TN. He is a professor Emeritus at the Quillen College of Medicine, ETSU. He is Board certified in IM and Pulmonary diseases. In addition to 43 years of practice in pulmonary and critical care medicine, he has served as a professor of Medicine and the Division Chief at the ETSU college of Medicine. During 1992-98, he also served as the assistant Dean of community health. Dr. J Mehta has received several outstanding awards for teaching and community service.

Dr. Mehta has published 8 books and more than 100 articles in medical journals. He has authored several chapters in medical textbooks. His lifelong interest in comparative religion led him to receive, MA degree in Eastern philosophy from HUA, Miami, Florida, and has presented many lectures on Bhagavat Gita and Upanishad. Dr. Mehta has trained many IM residents who became his fellowship students in Pulmonary and Critical care Medicine.

Kunj Patel, Undergraduate Student

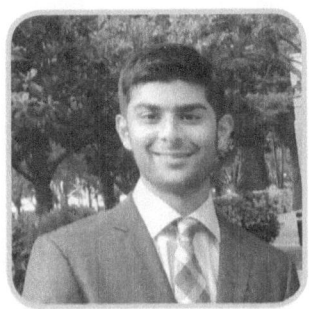

Kunj Patel is a third year Undergraduate student at the Illinois Institute of Technology and is pursuing his BS degree in Medicinal Chemistry with a minor in Premedical Studies. He is currently enrolled in the Lake Erie College of Medicine BS/DO early acceptance program. He currently pursuing undergraduate research in Computational Biochemistry and models biochemical systems. In the past, he had researched the application of Multifunctional Oxide Nanoparticles for medical imaging. Kunj currently holds ExCPT and PTCB pharmacy technician certifications. He is also CPR certified and holds several FEMA certifications related to emergency preparedness.

Indraine Ram, Ph. D.

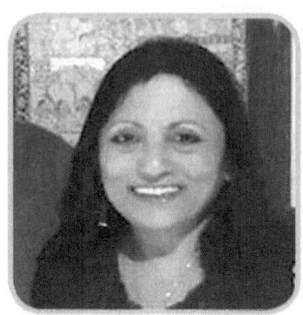

Dr. Indranie Gurusamy Ram, Ph.D. has a Ph.D. in Philosophy and has been an academic in the higher education sector for over 25 years. Dr. Ram is currently a semi-retired academic. She has been employed in both the Public and Private and Higher education sectors.

Dr. Ram was a Chief Operating Officer for Academic, Research and Quality Assurance at Pro-Active Public Services College for more than 10 years. She has recently retired from her full-time position and currently is an independent educational consultant. Dr. Ram's responsibilities in the Tertiary environment entailed Quality Assurance of academic and operational policies and procedures. She has written several training manuals and conducted training in various skills related and academic programs. She was on various committees while lecturing at the University including the Ethics Committee. She was contracted by the CHE (Council for Higher Education) to assess learning programs for accreditation of Higher Education Institutions in 2003.

Dr. Indranie Ram contributed to conference proceedings and presented papers at several local and international conferences. She presented a paper in Oxford at Mansfield College in September 2004; the Paper was entitled Moral Philosophy with Children. She presented a paper at the International Greek Society for Humanities Conference in May 2005; the Paper was entitled Morality and Consciousness. She presented a paper at the EMASA (Education Management Association of South Africa) Conference, Cape Town, March 2007; the Paper was entitled School and the World of Work, a Synergistic Alignment. She has published in **Phronimon** (Peer-reviewed journal); Vol 6 June 2005: Plato and Vedanta, DOE (Department of Education) accredited journal. She has authored "Management Philosophy toward an Ethical Worldview" (Chapter 8) in Bharat S. Thakkar, (Ed) 2020; Paradigm Shift in Management Philosophy: Future Challenges in Global Organizations; Publisher: Palgrave Macmillan. She has authored "An Analysis of a Unity of Cultural Perspectives to Achieve Global Business Success (Chapter 8) in Bharat S. Thakkar, (Ed) 2021; Culture in Global Businesses Addressing National and Organizational Challenges, Publisher: Palgrave Macmillan.

Dr. Indranie Ram as a semi-retired academic is passionate to make a contribution to Humanity and our Planet in respect of our responsibilities to assist society and global organizations to co-exist in a meaningful, pluralistic relationship with future decisions being based on Morality and the greater good for all.

Kadambari Ram, Ph.D.

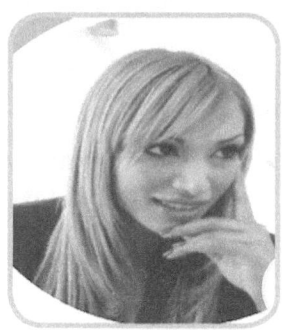

Dr. Kadambari Ram provides expert international vision and leadership with an international Ph.D. in information systems management, an international MBA from Purdue University, and an internationally recognized Certified Financial Officer (CFO) SA designation. Dr. Kadambari Ram's research involves complexity theory within the ambit of information systems and the application of evolutionary computing for understanding complex adaptive systems, specifically for addressing climate change as a critical leadership problem, game theory, and agent-based modeling and simulation.

As an expert in simulation modeling Dr. Kadambari Ram developed the resilience, robustness, sustainability, and adaptive-capacity (RRSA) simulation tool for assessing organizational contributions to climate change. Dr. Kadambari Ram is listed on the consultant roster for the United Nations Framework Convention for Climate Change (UNFCCC).

As an entrepreneur Dr. Kadambari Ram pioneered the combination of medical aesthetics and dentistry in Cape Town, South Africa holding the Zen Aesthetic™ and Zen Clinical™ trademarks in this sector. Dr. Kadambari Ram is the founding executive director of Zen Aesthetic Dental Spa, and the founding executive director of

Empirical Institute of Research. Dr. Kadambari Ram is an advocate of social change, specifically relating to the linkages between disease, climate change, and the consumption of animal derived products. Dr. Kadambari Ram's numerous accolades in music, combined with her practice of yoga, and academic research have produced an approach to leadership involving development of the self for service to society and the greater biosphere through a combination of techniques under the trademark Selphology™ for delivering these tools.

Kevin Sorbello, Ph.D.

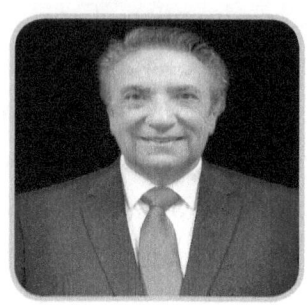

Dr. Sorbello is a part-time professor specializing in leadership and global supply chain management at Capella University and a full-time Manager of Training for a US government contractor. Dr. Sorbello is also a licensed Merchant Marine Chief Engineer of Gas Turbine, Steam, and Motor vessels of any horsepower. Dr. Sorbello also holds an M.A. in Management Philosophy from Walden University and an M.A. in National Security and Strategic Studies from the US Naval War College. He is also a certified instructor for Reliability Centered Maintenance and Root Cause Analysis, has led teams on several humanitarian support missions on the island of East Timor, and received the Arthur L. Johnson award for Inspirational Leadership by the US Navy League. Dr. Sorbello focuses on global business processes and development that include cultural awareness and inclusion, and virtual management. In addition to his qualitative study exploring the influences of subcultural perceptions on change success, he has contributed chapters to the *Paradigm Shift in Management Philosophy* and *Culture in Global Businesses*, both edited collections by Dr. Bharat Thakkar. He can be reached by email at kevin.sorbello@capella.edu.

Bharat S. Thakkar, Ph.D., Editor

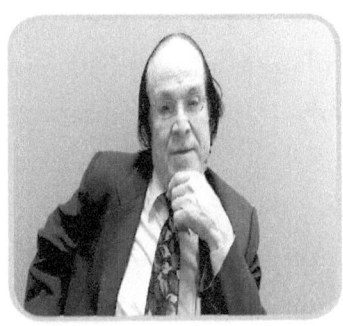

Dr. Thakkar received his M.S. and Ph.D. degrees from Illinois Institute of Technology. He had published and presented over thirty-five technical papers and holds two U. S. patents. In April 2018, January 2020, and December 2020, (Palgrave / McMillan Publisher), Dr. Thakkar edited three books, one on "The Future of Leadership": (ISBN: 978-3-319- 73870-3), "Paradigm Shift in Management Philosophy" (ISBN: 978-3-030-29709-1), and "Culture in Global Businesses" (ISBN: 978-3-030-60295-6) respectively. These books were designed to be used as textbooks in universities and reference books for professionals.

Since last twenty years Dr. Thakkar has been teaching MBA, DBA, and Ph.D. management courses in Chicago-area colleges and universities along with presentations at various workshops and conferences. In fall of 1997, Illinois Institute of Technology conferred Alva C. Todd Professorship upon Dr. Thakkar.

Dr. Thakkar has been engaged in the practice of reliability engineering and management over last thirty-five years of which last twenty-six years were spent with Lucent Technologies (formerly AT&T Bell Laboratories). He has published and presented over forty technical papers and holds two US patents.

Dr. Thakkar was involved in Graduate Business Curriculum development, teaching, recruiting, and scheduling courses at Argosy University for over six years. He had been Interim Chairman of the Department in 2009 till a permanent Chair was hired. His research interests are Leadership, Operations Management, Globalization, Complex Decision-making Tools and Techniques, Quantitative Research Methodology, and Systems Reliability Engineering and Management. Dr. Thakkar's interest in enriching community revolves around well-being of minority groups and making sure, no one is discriminated based upon nationality, race, color, creed, and religion. He is a firm believer in promoting diversity and harmony in his work environment and community where he lives.

Dr. Akesh, Thomas, MD

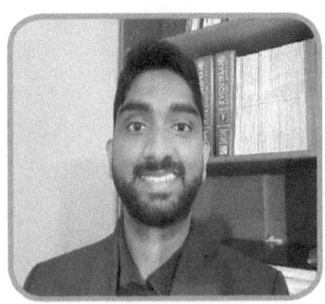

Dr. Akesh Thomas is a resident physician in Internal Medicine at East Tennessee State University Quillen College of Medicine. Akesh has a special interest in pulmonary medicine and health equity. Akesh has been in the frontlines of COVID care from the beginning of the COVID19 crisis in Tennessee. Akesh can be reached at thomasa16@ etsu.edu

FOREWORD

by Kevin Sorbello

I have always had a desire to understand how things work from the mechanical to the societal. Coupled with these interests was an innate desire to lead others in ways that helped them grow into skillful and self-confident members of society and the workforce. I am, at heart, a situational and transformational leader. I am also recognized as an expert in the fields of marine engineering, supply chain management and transformational leadership. My eclectic interests and hobbies include astrophysics, music, quantum mechanics, poetry, medicine, marine engineering, leadership theory, and its practical application across cultural lines.

I met Dr. Bharat Thakkar while I was a PhD student nearing the end of my thirty-two-year career as a merchant marine chief engineer and program manager in government service. Dr. Thakkar proved to be an excellent educator with extensive experience in similar areas of interest and who shared my love of poetry. I learned much about Dr. Thakkar while he served as my professor in leadership and long after while helping edit a few of his books of poetry. Much of what I learned was about the depth and breadth of his knowledge and experience across several subjects critical to understanding the business world and the technical and leadership challenges inherent in operating a successful business in a global market. Decade's worth of experience while serving as a merchant marine chief engineer traveling around the world exposed me to the various business and supply chain practices, leadership and management challenges, and cultural diversity issues not normally encountered by someone born in the US working for one or more globalized companies. Comparing this experience with Dr. Thakkar, born and educated in India, reinforced my understanding of these issues and further added to the respect I held for his unique skills and capabilities, particularly in the area of leveraging the knowledge, experience, and perspectives of others when addressing global business and leadership issues from multiple angles.

Dr. Thakkar has a talent for gathering and leveraging the knowledge, experience, and insights of experts in leadership and management. His efforts include a three-book series on leadership and management: *The Future of Leadership: Addressing Complex Global Issues* (2018) ISBN 978-3-319-73869-7, *Paradigm Shift in Management Philosophy: Future Challenges in Global Organizations* (2020) ISBN 978-3-030-29709, and *Culture in Global Businesses: Addressing National and Organizational Challenges* (2021) ISBN 978-3-030-60296-3. These three books (publisher: Palgrave/Macmillan) collectively address leadership and management evolution, issues, and challenges, offering scholarly insights, predictions, and recommendations from recognized experts with diverse backgrounds and experiences. Dr. Thakkar's ability to reach out, identify, and collect scholars who wish to collaborate on these topics is unique, and the fruit of his labors provide valuable information and perspectives to those leaders and managers who must face an ever-changing, ever-evolving landscape that continues to present unexpected challenges to businesses, large or small. This book, although not part of the previous trilogy on leadership and management, provides similarly valuable information and insights associated with the recent COVID-19 pandemic—an expected yet unanticipated event that presented new and unique challenges to business leaders on a global scale.

Experts in virology have been warning of a possible pandemic for decades, yet with plenty of time to prepare for what these experts considered inevitable, the world proved to be much unprepared from medical infrastructure, research, supply chain, social psychology, governmental policy, and business process perspectives. Regardless of the true source of the pandemic, its identification and the responses offered by governments around the world created chaos for social norms and processes on a scale previously unknown. Perhaps the most significant difference between this pandemic and previous pandemics is the interdependence and network structure of communication, supply chains, travel options, and speed of transmission across national and cultural lines. In an age accustomed to change happening at increasingly accelerated rates and nearly instantaneous communication, the pandemic disrupted nearly every aspect of business and personal life. Lockdowns, layoffs, business closures, and often conflicting policies and information created unique situations that could not be addressed with a single cure or methodology. Dr. Thakkar felt strongly that the next book should focus on the significant challenges that were created by the pandemic and offer insights and context to those who were in positions to address the problems created by this global disruption.

Similarly, this pandemic revealed the degree of unpreparedness of governments, businesses, and publicly and privately funded research regarding any significantly disruptive global event. The pandemic was a medical event, yet there are a host of other events that could create unique situations requiring a completely different set of responses. Earthquakes, eruptions, tidal waves, nuclear incidents, civil wars, global wars, meteor impacts, cyberattacks or ransomware affecting national or global infrastructures and services, and other as-yet-unidentified events could disrupt supply chains, labor availability, physical capabilities, and government policies in ways that could result in a complete collapse of any business or government's operations. It is hoped that those who read this book will gain insights from recent events that will help leaders and managers address current challenges and better prepare them for the next disruptive event.

According to a report published by Dell Technologies, authored by the Institute for the Future (IFTF) and a panel of 20 business, tech, and academic experts from around the world, 85% of the jobs that will exist in 2030 (only 9 years away at the time of this writing) have not yet been invented (SaLemi 2018). Even if this prediction is only partially correct, the implication is that advances in technology might require adapting to a new normal on a scale equivalent to a globally disruptive event. It is, therefore, critical that the lessons learned, the insights gleaned, and the experience gained from addressing issues created by the COVID-19 pandemic are applied in a way that prepares school, business, social, and governmental leaders for future disruptions, whether the result of another pandemic, environmental, social, or governmental disasters, or the aerated changes due to advances in technology. Returning to previous models of social and business norms is unrealistic. The changes in the way we go about our daily lives, operate businesses, elect our official representatives, provide products and services, and interface with one another are irreversible. Cultural lines continue to blur and divide into subcultural niches that can unite or divide us moving forward. How businesses deal with these realities will determine whether they will thrive or wither and disappear. Mass migrations, social distancing, vaccination mandates, lockdowns, virtual work environments, and new class structures must be addressed in previously unexpected ways. It is with this realization that Dr. Thakkar has brought together a collection of authors whose chapters present their perspectives, predictions, and recommendations for those who wish to succeed in this volatile landscape.

Reference

SaLemi, L. 2018. "85% of Jobs that will exist in 2030 haven't been invented yet." *LinkedIn*. https://www.linkedin.com/pulse/85-jobs-exist-2030-havent-been-invented-yet-leo-salemi.

PREFACE

Change Management of Global Businesses during a Pandemic Addressing COVID-19 Issues Affecting Human Race

by Bharat Thakkar

A pathogen measuring between 50 and 140 nanometers (nm) has shaken up our planet and its nearly eight billion inhabitants. When you consider that one nanometer is one-billionth of a meter, you begin to grasp how vulnerable our civilization is even to a nanoscale entity which is not technically considered alive unless it finds and resides in a living host cell. Coronavirus disease 2019 or COVID-19 is a SARS variant virus which, like other viruses, needs a host to thrive and multiply. We humans are that primary host in addition to possibly animals and birds.

It is not quite Third World War with its roots in biological warfare, but the consequences of the way the SARS CoV-2, as the coronavirus is called, has spread; it has mimicked many of the ways of biological warfare. Humans have lived with viruses for a very long time, ever since the human beings existed but even then, the realization that they cannot be seen or touched or smelled, yet they can be so lethal is frightening. If a science fiction writer in the medieval period visualized our world in the twenty-first century confronting something so extraordinary, he or she would have been probably declared a heretic and burned at the stake.

What is extraordinary about the SARS CoV-2, like all such outbreaks, is that it is so sudden and spreads so quickly. In a span of a few months since its first detection in Wuhan province of China in early 2019, the virus had the world in its deathly grip rapidly destroying societal balance across the globe. Apart from the obvious death and sheer physical suffering, the virus deeply affected personal relationships including individual's state of well-being. It hived off parents from children, husbands from wives, and families from families at one level. At another, it also destroyed marriages because of long periods of spouses being confined to their homes. Then there was the profound impact on the way offices functioned. Hundreds of millions of workers, if not more than a billion, had to be forced to stay home and work from there. That in turn led to the emergence of more sophisticated video conference technologies such as Zoom and Microsoft Teams. Just as there was a time once when photocopying was called Xeroxing, derived from its manufacturer Xerox, video conferencing became Zooming.

One of the most remarkable consequences of the pandemic has been that once it began to subside in early 2021, workers by the millions chose either not to return to work from the traditional office spaces or altogether left their jobs. However, toward the end of 2021, especially in the last week of November the virus mutated in a dramatic fashion in a new variant called omicron which the World Health Organization (WHO) designated a "variant of concern." On two important markers of transmissibility and severity of the disease the WHO said in the immediate aftermath of the mutation, it was not clear how worrisome the two were. The rise of this new variant out of South Africa yet again threw the world back into a period of uncertainty, even though by the middle of December 2021, only one death was attributed to the Omicron variant.

The virus upended politics in many parts of the world, including in America where the politics of the virus devoured the science of the virus and continues to do it over two years after it was first detected. Mask mandates caused deep parental divides across America with parents opposing the wearing of masks often getting into physical altercations with those insisting on it. School board meetings around America became a volatile battleground for political fights.

Who would have thought that a pathogen measuring in nanometers could so powerfully disrupt our world? This book attempts to look at the phenomenon from many different angles including how businesses around the world will have to manage this unprecedented but a long-lasting change.

The managers and leaders in business organizations are not sure what exactly is happening to their businesses in such an unpredictable and ever-changing toxic environment. The current COVID-19 pandemic has been a global stressor unprecedented in recent history. This book attempts to identify and provide the tools of change to help management to understand the complexity of the situation created by pandemic and how businesses and administrations might be able to minimize the impact of changes resulting from reactions to pandemic. Whether or not a Third World War has happened is a moot point, the effective change management strategies may be the only hope that neutralizing the issues and negative effects of the 2019-2022 pandemic is possible. This book provides methods that effectively address change management problems arising from the COVID-19 pandemic promoting innovation and adaptation to the creation of effective change management strategies that address unique business issues unprecedented in the modern business world.

Government and societal responses to the COVID-19 made virtual hostages of eight billion people from the end of 2019 through the beginning of 2022 by imposing stay-at-home orders, the shutting down of nonessential businesses, and an elevated fear of the unknown mortality associated with contact even between family members. Variants of the virus continued to threaten lives from the latter part of 2020 well into 2022 with subsequent confusion among the medical community and society at large on the efficacy of the existing vaccines against them.

The invention of PCR (Polymerase Chain Reaction) in 1983 was a game changer. Instead of waiting for viruses to grow naturally like in culture tests, PCR technique concentrates the DNA material from sample and rapidly multiplies tiny amounts of viral DNA exponentially in a series of heating and cooling cycles that can be automated and completed in less than an hour. The inventor of PCR, Kary Mullis, who won the Nobel Prize in Chemistry in 1993, argued that PCR was an effective way to identify the presence of viruses, but vehemently opposed using PCR to diagnose diseases: "PCR is a process that's used to make a whole lot of something out of something. It allows you to take a very miniscule amount of anything and make it measurable and then talk about it like it is important. PCR has certainly allowed public health authorities and the media around the world to talk about a new variant of Coronavirus like it's important, but how important is it really? The presence of the virus is not an indicator that someone has contracted the disease, especially since many people are naturally immune or asymptomatic, where the presence of a small amount of the virus might count the person as a case of infection.

By the time, this book is in print we will be in throws of the Omicron variant. If predictions by scientists and pundits come true, by end of 2022, coronavirus disease will become endemic from pandemic. Hopefully by then the jury will also be out on the use of PCR testing used as a gold standard to declare coronavirus as pandemic and more mortality threatening than it actually was.

This pandemic is more than just a medical challenge because it has been politicized by the media and government officials around the world. Media pundits in support of specific political ideologies routinely use it to promote their agendas by selecting data that supports their position, while leaving out or discrediting data that challenges it. Creating additional confusion and distrust in the media, medical experts, and government officials is the conflicting advice provided by medical experts, the centers for disease control (CDC), and public figures in the entertainment and sports industry. The emotional impact of such conflicting information has made good governance and business planning more difficult than any time in modern history. The ensuing battle between the reaction to the pandemic and politics is real, and few agree on any practical solutions. Businesses were ill prepared for such a change in their environment based on the reaction to a virus with a lower non-immunized mortality than other viruses exhibited in modern times. It was because all past episodes were not related to respiratory virus. This situation has left a gaping hole in plans to apply the existing portfolio of change management strategies that did not consider such extreme changes occurring in such a short time.

Corporations predicting exterior environmental changes that would result in losing profits and revenues use change management to adapt their business practices to bring their financials in control. However, at no time in the past hundred years have businesses been forced to shut down or allow remote support of their services to simply survive for such an extended period.

This pandemic has drawn attention to global health systems, the World Health Organization (WHO), the CDC, virologists, vaccine research and development, manufacturing, and distribution, and the introduction of expedited approval of vaccines that used genetic manipulation, splicing, and recombination techniques previously used only for research and development of genetically modified organisms for human consumption. The declining economies and public mistrust in authorities has reached unprecedented levels that further exacerbate business manager attempts at instilling confidence in workforce safety and approval to operate under strict and at times oppressive health guidelines. The damage to social norms and business practices created by the pandemic and governmental reaction or overreaction to the perceived threat is unprecedented. The actual toll of human suffering and educational disparities will most likely be disproportionate to the actual threat and remains to be seen. However, the impact to business, especially small and middle-sized businesses, may be far greater than predictions foretell if strategies to recover are not in place by the end of 2022.

It is understood and recognized that the mention of SARS and MERS which happened in last few decades is also historically meaningful in this book. The effects of the pandemic and the responses taken to reduce the lethality and spread of the virus, plus advances in technology and an accelerated shift dominated by social media platforms and virtual business models, may have created a quantum jump to certain future models designed to increase the level and number of remote workers. Predictions by business experts suggest there will not be a return, or at least a full return, to the old business model, yet this provides opportunities that could result in increased profit by leveraging decreases in overhead and travel costs, which is another strategic option available to business leaders moving forward.

Change management is the umbrella under which front-line management, teleworking, social media, empathic communication, and innovation during a crisis must be addressed in the COVID-19 era. Front-line managers are the group with the most connection to staff motivation, engagement, morale, and performance, and therefore, they need to be prepared for major social external changes such as COVID-19 and its demand on individuals within the organization as well as the organization as a whole. Although COVID-19 exemplified the urgent need for teleworking in the survival of organizations, teleworking is here to stay and will push the need to invest in reorganizing the managerial approach to accommodate methods compatible with working from the remote such as benefits and cultural change.

The COVID-19 outbreak, in particular, has highlighted the necessity for change management in the development of a comprehensive social media communication strategy in the time of a crisis. Organizations can no longer afford the effects of misinformation, scaremongering, or trivialization of organizational events, status, or needs. Under the change management umbrella, empathic communication and innovation during a crisis surfaced as high-priority skill needs. COVID-19 brought the need for the skill to communicate empathy openly and honestly to build trust in human interactions as an essential element of survival. Empathic communication has been emphasized in medical settings, but COVID-19 brought the realization of need infused into diverse communications in a broad range of interactions throughout organizations.

An additional high-powered tool during any change management process is innovation. Innovation means doing something differently than has been done before. Therefore, the more your business innovates, the more unique it becomes. Standing out from the pack helps ensure that your business can survive the new businesses flooding the market. With closures and social distancing, came the testing of innovation skills and viability of changes.

This book offers various solutions that minimize or leverage the impact and changes brought about by the pandemic by employing targeted change management strategies. My hope is to intellectually address the management and leadership issues in controlling and stemming the worldwide losses of business endeavors, and human resources within new economic environments through the application of strategic change management. Providing the history of pandemic or endemic was a good piece of work dating back to earlier available records.

It has been a confusing and chaotic ride with Covid-19 for everyone around the globe for more than two years . We have come a long way in trying to understand Covid-19. But a lot remains to be fathomed, including long Covid (Some people with COVID-19 have lingering symptoms for weeks or months after they begin to recover. You might know this as "long COVID." Experts have coined a new term for it: post-acute sequelae SARS-CoV-2 infection (PASC); fourth vaccine shot (2 regular and 2 booster shots) for elderly and citizens with underlying medical conditions; mixing of vaccines; effects of vaccines on our mind, body and soul, vaccine effectiveness period as well as vaccine mortality. I hope to cover these and other relevant issues in future publications thereby improving our collective understanding. While we have taken remarkable strides in understanding the Covid-19, there remains a great deal still to comprehend about its complexities. Your support has been my driving force in this onward journey. I hope you extend it.

In putting this volume together, I must thank Dr. Jayant Mehta, Dr. Rahul Patel, Dr. Aridaman K. Jain, Dr. Prince Emmanuel, and Dr. Kevin Sorbello for their advice and counseling. I thank Mr. Mayank Chhaya for the cover design concept for this book. He has been particularly resourceful in advising on matters of publisher selection and organizational aspects of this book. I must thank Dr. Lydia Daniels for writing Introduction for this book on a short notice. Finally, I wish to congratulate all authors of this volume who took on the challenge to think about COVID-19, an unusual phenomenon in recent times.

I also personally want to thank Ms. Harriet Fulton, Ms. Mary Flores, Elijah Rivers, Kaye Parsons and their associates from Xlibris Publishing Company for collaborating with me to realize this valuable contribution to recent pandemic and Change Management literature.

INTRODUCTION

by Lydia Daniels

The twenty-first century has brought a plethora of events which have dramatically increased the perception of instability, insecurity, and uncertainty around the globe, the most recently traumatic and deadly of which has been the COVID-19 pandemic. While the essence of the COVID-19 pandemic lies in the arena of a public health crisis, the resultant global effects encompass every phase of our lives: health, family, economy, technology, business, social interaction, education, employment, entertainment, livelihood, to name a few areas. Recognizing the complexity of the phenomena in our era, through foresight and ingenuity, the editor Bharat S. Thakkar has identified and brought together highly recognized experts in their disciplines to untangle the complexity and together bring us a realistic view of the issues and dynamics of the era from which we might seek to contribute to the greater good on an individual and professional path forward. In an environment of misinformation and disinformation, this book of wisdom and inspiration is a must-read for all seekers on the journey to a utopian world.

The inspirational and informative chapters in this book include:

- Dr. Kadambari Ram's explanation of the complexity of the COVID-19 pandemic, the link between pandemics and catastrophic collapse of global systems, and change management.

- Dr. Sorbello's chronology of the COVID-19 pandemic and exploration of what changes and challenges lie ahead for change managers in the current and post-pandemic world.

- Dr. Brahmbhatt's definition and review of the gig economy and the COVID- 19 impact;

- Dr. McIntosh's report on the economic impact of the pandemic and suggestions for survival and recovery.

- Dr. Joshi's collection of global research on how technology startups and technology entrepreneurship are likely to be impacted by COVID-19 and insights for the future of technology entrepreneurship in India.

- Dr. Gurusamy Ram's analysis of the application of strategic collaboration and cooperation by the leaders and the scientific community during the COVID-19 pandemic and examination of how priorities within the scientific community were established.

- Dr. Thomas and Dr. Mehta's review of healthcare workers' experiences during the coronavirus pandemic through case studies and the lessons learned in preparation for future epidemics of this magnitude.

- Mr. Patel's in-depth explanation of how the virus works and how this knowledge can inform people and allow them to analyze which measures should be taken to combat the COVID-19 pandemic.

- Dr. Casati and Dr. Sorbello's introduction of a new approach to change management through quantum computing technology; and

- Mr. Chhaya's sharing of a journalist's perspective on the interrelatedness of world poverty, global health systems, supply chains, jobs, and societal balance in a pandemic world.

The depth and detail of each chapter portend the knowledge and rigorous exploration of each author to provide a comprehensive framework from many angles to grasp the complexity of a post-pandemic world as a foundation from which to move forward with understanding and knowledge for future world-building. Thanks are extended to Dr. Thakkar for identifying the need to bring this broad scope of factual information into a one-book compilation, finding the contributing authors to share their scholarly research and expertise, and for his diligent editorship. My deep appreciation is also extended to Dr. Sorbello for the foreword.

Finally, the theme of this book is change management. I am reminded of the following quote by Mahatma Gandhi (1869–1948), "You must be the change you want to see in the world."

CHAPTER 1

COVID-19 Pandemic Complexity: The Tipping Point for Decision-Making

by Kadambari Ram

Abstract

Although the term complexity is widely used in nonacademic literature and daily life, the true definition of complexity as a theory in the academic sense is scientific and multidisciplinary in nature. In "Complexity: The tipping point for leadership," (Ram 2017) a projection toward labor and financial collapses associated with world epidemics or pandemics is directly linked to climate change and its deleterious consequences. This chapter serves to elucidate the misalignment of the linear methods, protocols, and policies with the decision-making needs of a complex problem such as the COVID-19 pandemic and the link to the catastrophic collapse of global systems. The need to implement a framework of decision-making for complex problems is emphasized in this chapter. The framework for resilience, robustness, and sustainability for improving adaptive capacity to complex problems such as global pandemics, climate change, and catastrophic collapse of global systems, within the ambit of change management (Ram), is more pertinent now than ever before in its urgency for implementation.

Keywords: complexity, COVID-19 pandemic, decision-making, catastrophic collapse, adaptive capacity, change management.

1.0 The Link between Pandemics and Catastrophic Collapse of Global Systems

1.1 Understanding Types of Collapse

Collapse in the literature is a term used to define the behavior of a system under strain due to resource depletion such that there is an overshoot of the carrying capacity of that system and decline or complete disappearance of the civilizations, empires, nations, or cultures that depend upon those resources for survival. Societies that succumb to collapse also demonstrate extreme economic stratification between wealthy and poor or elites and commoners (Motesharrei et al. 2014). Collapse is an endogenous process, meaning that it is the result of behavior within the system, such as farming to unsustainable levels. Take the example of a forest that is being used for its wood. If there are one hundred trees in the forest, the closer the logger gets to cutting down one hundred trees before new trees have grown, the closer the forest gets to overshooting its carrying capacity and collapse as a forest ecosystem. This type of collapse is triggered by a scarcity in nature of natural resources when the natural system does not recover and is known as a Type-N collapse such as the collapse of Easter Island and the resulting obliteration of its population.

In addition to Type-N collapses throughout history, we have had pivotal and recurring societal collapses triggered by the scarcity of workers resulting in population and wealth collapses or Type-L collapses. Both Type-N and Type-L collapses are evidenced by the rise, decline, and in some cases, complete disappearance of great civilizations and cultures throughout the world, such as the Roman, Minoan, Mycenaean, Sumerian, Akkadian, Assyrian, Babylonian, Achaemenid, Seleucid, Parthian, Sassanid, Umayyad, Abbasid, Mesopotamian, Hittite, Harrapan, Mauryan, Gupta, Khmer, Zhou, Han, Tang, Song, Mayan, Teotihuacan, Monte Alban, Cahokia, Pueblo, Hohokam, Tiwanaku, the decline of Zimbabwe, and the collapse of Easter Island. Many of these historical cases of collapse demonstrated the characteristics of ecological strain and economic stratification. The diversity of the societies that have collapsed indicated a global distribution ranging from Rome to India, to China, to southwest US countries, and to Africa. These are the societal collapses that we know of because these empires, cultures, and civilizations had sufficient complexity to produce written records or archeological evidence of their existence. So, the possibility exists that there could be other collapses which we are not aware of due to the lack of documentation or archaeological findings.

Many of these collapsed civilizations followed a boom-bust cycle over long periods before they finally completely disappeared. According to Motesharrei et al., the boom-bust cycle of collapse can extend over three hundred–five hundred years and can result in a decline of 30%–60% of a region's population. The recurrent trend of Type-N and L collapses throughout history and their global distribution, despite the complexity, sophistication, or creativity of the civilizations that declined, points to the susceptibility of our current situation. Despite our technological advancements, our continued reliance on the production of hydrocarbons by the oil and gas industry despite their deleterious effects on the environment, farming to unsustainable levels, the visible global economic stratification between wealthy and impoverished, climate change, global warming, and the COVD-19 pandemic are concerns for both Type-N and L collapses on a global scale, comprising the perfect storm for catastrophic collapse of global systems, including the traditional Keynesian economic and financial systems (Ram 2020).

1.2 Catastrophic Collapse

Catastrophes such as hurricane Katrina, various tsunamis, crises of civil unrest such as that which occurred in Kwa-Zulu Natal South Africa in July 2021, September 11, and the COVID-19 pandemic are scenarios that provide insight into how nation-states might improve their ability to proactively prevent and prepare for crises and disaster, rather than merely responding when the event is already underway. The canary in a coal mine is an appropriate metaphor to illustrate how devastating the inability to read signals from the environment might be (Kuecker 2007). In this metaphor, the coal miner's canary is huffing and gasping for air, signaling to the coal miner that the oxygen levels in the mine are catastrophically low, but stemming from his compounded denial of the criticality of the situation, the coal miner's belief that the canary is still alive and well, prevents him from evacuating the mine in time, and they both die. In this metaphor, the canary huffing and puffing could have been used as an early detection mechanism for the depletion of oxygen in the mine.

This problem of how people view reality through a deeply deceptive lens of denial is associated with public policies that are driven by faulty direct feedback models of productivity and economic output (Kuecker 2020). For example, Solow (1957) found that the relationship between production, labor, and capital did not reflect historical data for US economic output in the 1950s unless the function was multiplied by a factor of $A(t)$, a quantitative measurement of how technological advancements translated into productivity. The original equation $Y = L^a K^b$, where Y is production or economic output, L is labor, K is capital, and the exponents a and b are elasticities was then multiplied by $A(t)$, also known as the *Solow residual* or *total factor productivity*. According to the *total factor productivity* principle, technological improvement would always mitigate resource depletion thereby maintaining productivity. The flaws in this approach should be evident as stabilization is only one aspect of living systems, but the other attributes of learning, growth, and diversification are absent in the function. Societal behavior influenced by public policies built around such direct feedback models will fall drastically behind the moving reality which includes elements of stabilization, learning, growth, and diversification at a minimum. Kelly (1994) rightfully argued for a simulation artificial evolutionary model to capture the complexities of living systems.

1.3 Models and Reality

This work builds on a previous essay I wrote entitled "Complexity: The Tipping Point for Leadership" (Ram 2017) in which I discussed how future leaders should be able to use the appropriate tools for the prediction of future catastrophic events to prepare for them and respond accordingly. Prediction is after all the holy grail of science, and when we have developed a rule of law, we refer to it as an exact science as it can theoretically, perfectly predict the outcome of a system based on its inputs. For example, if you want to know how fast to drive your car to get to a certain place in a given time, you can use the equation

$s = d/t$, where s is speed, d is distance, and t is time. This is one of the simplest examples of perfect linear predictability assuming all else remains constant. The assuming all-else-remains-constant part is where things get tricky. For the $s = d/t$ equation to accurately predict the speed you should drive at, you must be driving from A to B on a road with constant friction, no speed bumps or obstacles, no traffic lights, no traffic, or any other cars in fact. You must have a perfectly unobstructed path that is constantly smooth throughout the journey for the equation's perfect prediction to work. You might say, "Well, that is obviously not a very useful tool for prediction if the conditions for the journey are so far from reality." When you think about it like this, it becomes obvious why some models fail in reality. A scientist might add variables to the $s = d/t$ equation for road friction, traffic, changes in routes, etc., so the equation becomes a model that better fits reality, and the prediction results become more useful. The model might be used to develop smart phone applications that guide you on the road or predict how long it will take you to get to the supermarket. Now that makes more sense you say. Yes, simply put, models become better at prediction the more complex they are within reason. For example, Ansell and Gash (2008) developed the *contingency model* of collaborative governance and found the process of collaboration to be of a complex nature, exhibiting characteristics of complexity theory such as path dependence and sensitive dependence on initial conditions.

Complex models are built in different ways. Due to the number of variables and the multitude of possible interactions and scenarios, computer simulations are used to test scenarios for complex models. Similarly, I developed the resilience, robustness, sustainability, and adaptive-capacity (RRSA) model for leaders as a predictive tool for complex problems such as climate change, global warming, and epidemics or pandemics. It is a complex model for complex problems.

The variables resilience, robustness, sustainability, and adaptive capacity are discussed below; however, further detail on how the model works, how it was developed, the methodology, and theoretical underpinnings are available in my dissertation (Ram 2017).

1.4 Resilience

On the construct of resilience, the literature points to several attempts at defining resilience within different contexts; however, this stimulation study uses a highly integrated approach to social, economic, ecological, and technological systems, the intersection of which are socioeconomic systems, socio-ecological systems (SESs), and socio-technological systems (STSs) respectively. This integrated approach aligns with the approach of *Disturbance as Opportunity* (Folke 2006) for the purpose of defining factors and their interaction when modeling SESs and organizational resilience to climate change and stresses the integration of five types of capital namely social, economic, human, physical, and natural capital to the resilience of SESs (Mayunga 2007) requiring a cross-scalar perspective including social norms, values such as trust, networks, air, water, and soil (Bahadur et al. 2010).

The construct of resilience originally derives from ecological studies in the 1960s and early 1970s on predator-prey dynamics in relation to ecological stability theory (Holling 1973). In recent literature, Oliver et al. (2015) defined ecological resilience in terms of a system's ability to recover after a disturbance and maintain its adaptive capacity by resisting regime shifts. However, certain ecosystems such as tundra, boreal forest, mountains, Mediterranean-type ecosystems, mangroves and salt marshes, coral reefs, and the sea-ice biomes are particularly vulnerable to an increase in temperatures of 2 - 3 degrees Celsius as indicated by statistics related to degradation and extinction of species, thereby supporting the argument for ecosystem management as a resilience tool for mitigation against climate change impacts and complete collapse of the global ecosystem (Munang et al. 2013). Munang et al. aimed to clarify the central role of ecosystem management as a resilience tool in climate change adaptation and disaster risk reduction, discussed ad hoc initiatives driven by ecosystem-based adaptation strategies, the need for greater effort and collaboration concerning ecosystem management, and presented several benefits and advantages pertaining to the use of ecosystem-based adaptation strategies. Munang et al. concluded that the benefits and advantages of ecosystem management met the needs associated with UNFCCC priorities and the Hyogo Framework for Action, albeit requiring appropriate policy and action.

1.5 Resilience Management

On resilience management, Folke et al. (2005) noted that the costs of collaboration and conflict resolution might be lowered via the emergence of *bridging organizations*. Thus, the latter supports self-organization by enabling legislation and governmental policies for co-management of adaptive capacity efforts. Theoretically, the authors used a SESs approach based on the move from assessments using the maximum sustainable yield of individual species to the management of ecological processes. The work of Folke et al. resonated with that of Lemos et al. (2013) in that the authors observed the counterproductive effects of specific adaptive capacity efforts on the generic adaptive capacity of a system by using the mobilization of Belizian coastal fisherman as an example. The operationalization of adaptive governance was therefore proposed through adaptive co-management of systems, for which four essential features of SESs were presented. Ergo adaptive management, in contrast to conventional management, is the conceptualization that policies be treated as hypotheses and management actions are the experiments that test those hypotheses. This approach to adaptive management is both practical and methodological, serving as a topic for further examination within the field of organizational resilience and drawing attention to the intersection between resilience and adaptive capacity.

Similarly, a sustain-centric management paradigm presents several significant operationalization challenges to organizations. As the literature points out that an open systems view of resilience is empirically untapped, a lacuna exists for a consistent conceptualization of organizational resilience for practical and research purposes (Linnenluecke & Griffiths, 2010). In response to this gap, Linnenluecke and Griffiths outlined the main aspects of organizational resilience, discussing resilience and adaptive cycles. A valid contribution to the intersection between resilience and adaptive capacity was the insight that organizational requirements for coping with major disturbances exceed those for overcoming minor ones, thereby exceeding the thresholds for adaptation. The authors observed that the coping range of an organization might be important for statistically or objectively understanding the extremities of resilience.

Linnenluecke and Griffiths (2010) discussed climate change, extreme weather conditions, and the disastrous consequences therewith associated, provided examples using real cases, and developed a resilience framework for the study of organizational adaptation to climate change because an approach of economic factors of competition to the former lacks the necessary tools to provide a thorough understanding. Because of the economic factors approach, past methods of coping with sudden changes have included risk and crisis adaptation mechanisms. These mechanisms are aimed at mitigating the consequences of disruptions such as strikes, changes in demand and competition, accidents, etc.

However, the uncertainty and potentially disastrous consequences associated with climate change and extreme weather conditions are unprecedented. Therefore, the goal of the resilience framework is to facilitate organizational development of resources and capabilities that mitigate the disastrous consequence of organizational collapse because of climate change and weather extremes.

1.6 Robustness

The construct of resilience as it applies to networks within the field of information systems management directly informs this simulation study and is closely related to the construct of robustness in the literature. Watts' (2014) conceptualization of organizational robustness affirms the notion that authors use the terms robustness and resilience interchangeably, albeit incorrectly. The need to define the term robustness for constructing a simulation model calls for close inspection of the parameters, if any, and theories that apply. Watts opined that an organization's robustness, which involves the ability to allocate resources, innovate, adapt, and solve problems, is related to its organizational structure. The finding that robustness is a feature of a complex organization, operationalized by the prevention of failure on the one hand and preparation for its inevitability on the other directly informed my choice of robustness as an independent variable for this study and lead to the derivation of my hypothesis that robustness is required of organizations in order to adapt to climate change strategic objectives, supported by the pertinent example of the Internet, which is a networked system requiring robustness in order to survive unpredictable breakdowns.

Ay et al. (2012) argued that guided self-organization (GSO) pertains to the construct of robustness as it applies to network structure.

They defined self-organization as the transition of a system into an organized form in the absence of centralized control or an external agent, drawing attention to the seemingly paradoxical nature of the term, *guided self-organization* (GSO), and addressed this contradiction using optimal path formation within artificial ant colonies. Ay et al. highlighted the emergence of organized behavior because of interactions between agents and their environment in the absence of an overarching blueprint or design and clarified the difference between an implicit effect (i.e., change in the agent's decision-making mechanism) and an explicit effect (i.e., change to the environment).

Perception-action loops of embodied systems relating to GSO may be of value to my simulation. Viewing organizational resilience, robustness, and sustainability (RRS) through the lens of GSO provides a novel approach for modeling organizational RRS and the potential emergent behaviors that may result (Ay et al. 2012). Furthermore, the optimization principle mentioned by Ay et al. suggested that exploration emerges because of optimizing information gain rather than because of behavior randomization modelling. Thus, the cognitive aspect or embodied cognition among multiple agents of modelling emergence was emphasized and should be examined for further research. Of relevance was the perspective that living beings are information-processing systems and that an evolutionary advantage can be gained via the optimization of these processes. If the contention that surviving climate change is an evolutionary advantage holds, then mitigation of climate change may be operationalized through optimization of the information processes relating to living beings. The authors discussed the application of this method using the dynamical systems approach to robot control, stating that the learning rules derived from maximum PI may be used as a tool for self-organization of behavior in complex robotic systems, ergo may be used to guide the behavior of agents in this simulation study.

Gershenson (2011) discussed random Boolean networks (RBNs) as self-organizing systems to examine how the changes in nodes and connections affect the global network dynamics and discussed eight different methods for guiding the self-organization of RBNs with emphasis on guiding the RBN toward the critical dynamical regime. In slight contrast to the principles of GSO, a self-organizing system is described as one in which the elements interact, thereby dynamically producing a global pattern or behavior; a global pattern is produced from local interactions. Furthermore, Gershenson mentioned that any system can, in principle, be described as self-organizing, thereby prompting the question of when does it become useful to describe a system as self-organizing? Gershenson adequately answered this question by clarifying that self-organization becomes useful when there are at least two levels of description present (e.g., behaviors and individuals; teams and organization).

Gershenson's (2011) work is relevant to further research on modelling organizational resilience, robustness, and sustainability (RRS) from the perspective that the properties and advantages of the critical regime, which is the phase transition between the ordered and dynamical phases, apply to life, computation, adaptability, evolution, and robustness. Gershenson further recommended the application of the guidance methods of RBNs to engineering systems with features of the critical regime, as well as the study of how living systems evolved via natural selection. For my simulation study, I have conceived the organization as an embodied system, the properties of which can be easily interpreted through information dynamics, ergo organizational adaptability to climate change because RRS can be viewed as an embodied engineering system.

2.0 Emergence and Self-Organization for Robust Systems

Related to the work of Prokopenko and Gershenson (2014) about describing science using a nonreducing language, albeit for the purposes of GSO, Polani et al. (2013) elucidated the difference between emergence and self-organization using information theory and graph theory and an example of particles self-organizing devoid of any emergent pattern-like behavior. Polani et al. framed GSO as a set of principles that apply to the process of an organization across scales and contexts using the examples of a slime mold approach to the bio-development of motorways in the Netherlands, and ant-based algorithms with local optimization for community detection in large-scale networks, which shed light on the use of biological analogs for modelling networks, thereby substantiating the initial choice of cellular automata for this simulation study.

2.1 Evolutionary Robust Systems

Whitacre and Bender (2010) clarified the link between robustness and fitness of a system by discussing robustness within the context of evolution. Whitacre and Bender postulated that living systems display two desirable characteristics, namely, robustness and innovation; borrowing from biological taxonomy, the definition of phenotypic variability serves as a proxy for evolvability of a system. Whitacre and Bender shed light on the limitations of Darwin's principles of evolution for systems of unbounded complexity with the goal of developing a modern theory for the evolvability of unbounded complex systems based on the requirement of robustness using degeneracy, which is the partial redundancy of functions or capabilities of components in a system.

Whitacre and Bender (2010) applied biological taxonomy to computational requirements for modelling systems, evidenced by the phenotype attractor, and used a protein model consisting of genetically specified proteins to illustrate the concept of degeneracy as applied to modelling. Further discussion of the fitness landscape, neutral network, one-neighborhood and evolvability, robustness, and the fitness landscape exploration elucidated the degree to which design principles affect system evolvability. Whitacre and Bender clarified the link between robustness and evolvability of a system, ergo applied to this simulation study, an organization that is robust to climate change, or demonstrates a high degree of adaptability, must also be evolvable. These concepts have computational implications for modelling which when interpreted using information dynamics are relevant and necessary for modelling RRS.

2.2 Sustainability

The constructs of resilience, adaptive capacity, and robustness have been discussed within the contexts of social, ecological, technological, and their intersecting systems and may be applied to the phenomenon of climate change across all contexts, underpinned by the fact that industrial, social, and ecological systems are closely intertwined, calling for a comprehensive systems approach for effective decision-making regarding global sustainability (Fiksel 2006). Fiksel explored several questions aimed at providing guidance for future research and initiatives toward sustainability using a qualitative multi-case study approach and acknowledged the use of dynamic modelling techniques such as biocomplexity, system dynamics, and thermodynamic analysis by researchers to study the effects of climate change on ecological and human systems. Furthermore, resilience was discussed as a necessary quality of complex adaptive systems with the

US Environmental Protection Agency (EPS) incorporating the design of sustainable systems into their strategy.

While the construct of sustainability is interwoven in the literature on constructs already reviewed, it is necessary to include the triple-bottom-line (TBL) and triple value models as innovative frameworks that capture the nuances of sustainable systems, involving the flows between industrial, societal, and environmental systems (Elkington 1994, Fiksel et al. 2014, Slaper and Hall 2011). Slaper and Hall discussed Elkington's TBL model, which extended the traditional measurements of profits (i.e., return on investment and shareholder value to include environmental and social imperatives). Thus, the TBL model constitutes people, the planet, and profit as bottom-line contributors, thereby also referred to as the 3Ps. Slaper and Hall reviewed the TBL concept and its application for business, policymakers, and economic development practitioners and elucidated that defining the TBL is not where the difficulty lies but rather in measuring it. As such, the TBL was developed in response to the struggle involved with measuring sustainability and the 3Ps, ergo an associated strength of the TBL is that no universal index or standard measures exist. Instead a general framework may be applied to different entities based on various needs. As stakeholders determine TBL measures, depending on the level of entity, type of project, and geographic scope, the TBL framework may be adapted to either narrow or broad scopes. Slaper and Hall presented several traditional TBL economic, environmental, and social measures discussed variations of TBL measurement and dissected how businesses, nonprofits, and governmental entities might use the TBL with regard to each of the 3Ps or the economic, social, and environmental dimensions, including the importance of ecological stewardship.

Similarly, the triple value model involves identification of the value pathways in three types of capital assets, namely industrial economic capital, social and human capital, and natural capital, which are described and discussed in terms of motivations for adopting the approach and the results of its application (Fiksel et al. 2014). However, the relation of this approach to the triple-bottom-line approach, at least from a theoretical perspective was not mentioned. The application of the RRS model from this simulation study might be facilitated via the use of a triple-bottom-line or triple-value model.

Relating the construct of sustainability to policy and decision-making within a sub-Saharan context, Götz and Schäffler (2015) described ecological challenges facing the Gauteng City-Region, symptomatic of past political decisions to externalize environmental costs to future generations. Götz and Schäffler drew attention to the weak implementation of green economy strategies such as the Developmental Green Economy Strategy (2010) and the Green Strategic Programme (2011) in favor of continued industrial-policy style decision-making and the consequences thereof and discussed the Gauteng Green Strategic Programme (GGSP) within the Gauteng City-Region (GCR), outlining the major ecological issues of the GCR, such as acid mine drainage (AMD), variable rainfall patterns, high GHG emissions, poor air quality and high resource consumption in addition to socioeconomic challenges such as urban sprawl resulting from apartheid geographies, and the dependence of industries on cheap coal-fired electricity. Götz and Schäffler elucidated that the GGSP was developed in response to a massive economic downturn involving the loss of 250,000 jobs (6% of employment) between 2008 and 2010. The lack of implementation of GGSP objectives and goals clearly demonstrates the importance of political decision-making, governance, institutional support, and organizational capacity to operationalize strategy. Despite a well-defined mandate and existing programs for supporting green economic efforts, no progress has been made. Götz and Schäffler attributed this lack of progress to a common policy implementation problem embedded in cross-departmental cooperation challenges and a set of governmental conundrums, which they discussed in detail.

The work of Anderies et al. (2013) is of relevance to affecting sustainable global change. Anderies et al. noted that sustainability has become an accepted concern for organizational executives who do not possess the necessary tools or knowledge for its successful initiation. Additionally, the distinction between resilience, robustness, and sustainability was discussed in terms of their alignment for global change, thus substantiating the use of sustainability as an independent variable for this simulation study. Several pertinent examples were provided in support of the plausibility of sustainable actions at the individual level, be it firm, organizational, or other entity derailing sustainability at the global level or at the system level. Therefore, a key element for this study, derived from the work of Anderies et al. is the necessary distinction between the individual level of sustainable action and the global or systemic level thereof.

2.3 Sustainable Technology

Amemiya-Ramírez (2014) clarified the use and definition of sustainable technology, having no negative impact on the environment, society, the economy, or other technological systems and carrying out an assessment of sustainable technologies using hard and soft system analyses, both quantitative and qualitative in nature, respectively. Amemiya-Ramírez used a system dynamics modelling methodology and information on shale gas extraction as an alternate solution to the energy crisis of the 1970s to assess whether shale gas is a sustainable energy source and consequently provided a definition of sustainable societies, economies, environments, and technologies, explaining that aspects of the definition of sustainability are quantitative or measurable while other aspects are qualitative. Amemiya-Ramírez concluded that the production and use of shale gas contribute significantly to greenhouse gas (GHG) emissions with high water consumption involved in the extraction process, ergo shale gas was found to be an unsustainable energy source using system dynamics and simple modelling techniques.

2.4 Sustainability Management

The construct of sustainability as it applies to management is often framed in the literature within the context of social responsibility. For example, the ISO26000 standard formalizes the need for guidance on social responsibility and states, "An organization's performance in relation to the society in which it operates and to its impact on the environment has become a critical part of measuring its overall performance and its ability to continue operating effectively" (International Organization for Standardization [IOS] 2015, 2). Furthermore, ISO26000 was articulated as a mindset to be applied at all levels of the organization, such as planning, execution, and stakeholder interaction for right action, including the seven principles of social responsibility and their application to core subjects.

ISO26000 (2015) brought light to the fact that society's consumption outstrips the world's bio-capacity to regenerate by approximately 30%, thereby requiring organizational attention and further revealed in a study conducted in 2008 that social responsibility constituted the second leading force of change in quality. ISO26000 conceptualized organizational success as the dual objective of achieving sustainability through social impact and bottom-line growth. Furthermore, an integral characteristic of social responsibility was the willingness to include environmental and social considerations into decision-making and the accountability thereof.

2.5 Adaptive Capacity

As previously mentioned, closely linked to the construct of resilience is the construct of adaptive capacity, Nelson et al. (2007) framed the resilience approach as being systems-oriented with adaptive capacity serving as a core feature of social-ecologically resilient systems. Nelson et al. highlighted the role of robustness and adaptation in the conceptualization of resilience and the usefulness of resilience as a framework for analyzing adaptation processes and identification of appropriate policy responses. Additionally, the inherent characteristics of resilience were deemed to be consistent and capable of absorbing disturbances across scales (Nelson et al.). As such Nelson et al. distinguished between adaptation in the environmental change literature and adaptation within a resilience framework context, discussing the components of adaptation in detail. Nelson et al.'s description of adaptive capacity as a core precondition for a system to be able to adapt to perturbations feeds into my research and is supportive of the conceptual framework used for my model. The detail provided on the relationship between the characteristics, processes, and outcomes of an adaptive system is further useful for the purposes of modelling resilience. The contributions of Nelson et al.'s resilience framework are of particular relevance to my study, including descriptions of states, thresholds, surprise, and trade-offs in resilience and adaptiveness.

Engle (2011) addressed the role of adaptive capacity and how it relates to literature in the fields of resilience, vulnerability, sustainability, and the management thereof, articulating that there are few efforts concerned with the evaluation of adaptive capacity across resilience and vulnerability frameworks. As such adaptive capacity was defined as a prerequisite for leadership and organizational success in addition to the recommendations presented by the IPCCC (Engle). Furthermore,

Engle distinguished between different types of adaptation, clarifying the point that the complexity of adaptation is illustrated through maladaptation. In other words, adaptation is not linearly positive. Engle clarified the usefulness of adopting coupled SES as the unit of analysis in resilience research to understand the way mechanisms fit together within and across systems, which relates to interactions and emergence. Engle clarified the caveat for translating the construct of resilience into practice by discussing the role of adaptive capacity in resilience literature and how the former relates to vulnerability.

2.6 Adaptive Management and Governance

Of value to a discussion going forward on organizational adaptive capacity was the insight provided by Engle (2011) on the significant role of institutions, governance, and management in determining a system's ability to adapt to climate change. As such, the former bodies play a vital role in the redistribution of power and contributing to solving the justice issues intrinsic to the climate change debate, pointing to recent emphasis in the literature on adaptive management (AM) and adaptive governance (AG) research, which stresses realignment of decision making to the ecological scale. A key takeaway from Engle's work was the insight that the building of adaptive capacity is rooted in organizational theory but better suited for policy application through the coupled SES paradigm, appropriately viewed through the lenses of resilience and vulnerability.

Reeves and Deimler (2011) framed adaptability as a competitive advantage for organizations and outlined four organizational capabilities that facilitate adaptation. Reeves and Deimler opined that traditional approaches to strategy only apply to stable environments and that a rapidly changing and unpredictable world requires a different set of capabilities. According to Reeves and Deimler, these second-order capabilities foster rapid adaptation resulting in sustainable competitive advantage.

3.0 The Role of Technology

Reeves and Deimler (2011) discussed the role of technology in acquiring adaptability, specifically for experimental purposes within the context of testing services and products. The authors claimed that adaptable companies use experimentation to a greater degree than their competitors. Additionally, strategy follows organization in adaptive companies, which were conceived to withstand failure than those that are not adaptive. In other words, adaptive companies were found to be more robust to failure than their competitors because of dispersed and decentralized decision-making following a bottom-up rather than top-down approach. Reeves and Deimler's perspective that organizational adaptation to the environment, specifically to climate change, requiring robustness is relevant to this study and directly informs the choice of robustness as an independent variable for modelling adaptive capacity.

Lemos et al. (2013) argued that improved asset development, institutional access, and an awareness of institutional inequalities reduce vulnerability through a combination of policies and interventions thereby building adaptive capacity. Lemos et al. reviewed the literature pertaining to adaptive capacity, using the IPCC's categorization of the determinants of adaptive capacity as the basis of their paper aimed at understanding the factors that make human, social, and political systems less vulnerable to climate-related phenomena, using a conceptual foundation of adaptive capacity as generic on the one hand and specific on the other. Lemos et al. cited two cases, namely disaster risk reduction in Bangladesh and the governance and adaptive capacity of the Brazilian water sector. The second case aptly illustrated how stakeholder participation and integration can result in deleterious effects by reducing adaptive capacity, ergo indicating that specific and generic adaptive capacity efforts are not always positively related. Lemos et al. drew attention to the differentiation between specific and generic adaptive capacity, specifically their nonlinear relationship highlighted the inherent complexity of adaptive capacity. Nevertheless, an empirical analysis of this relationship was lacking in the literature and serves as an area for further research.

3.1 Adaptive Capacity and Climate Change

McEvoy et al. (2013) used a conceptual framework derived from studies on adaptation that are framed by the construct of resilience and included the effects of climate change and the difference in temporal and spatial scales of its problems in their discussion. McEvoy et al. opined that climate change is still in an embryonic stage of development, thus emphasizing the importance of *framing* the research and distinguishing between meta, conceptual, and operational types of frames for this purpose. McEvoy et al. proposed that the social framing of adaptation is necessary for collaborative processes, highlighting that differences in opinions might complicate decision-making. Thus, the implications of resilience as a frame for climate change adaptation were discussed for policy and practice (McEvoy et al.). Although resilience was an emergent frame for climate change adaptation, combining the use of both top-down and bottom-up approaches within an Australian context, the concepts associated with climate change and resilience can be thought of as universal; therefore, the conclusion that resilience is important for policy development in Australia, particularly relating to sustainable communities, is thought to be generalizable to all SESs within the literature.

4.0 Catastrophes, Disasters, and System Collapses through the Lens of RRSA

The constructs of resilience, robustness, sustainability, adaptive capacity, and climate change are often discussed in the literature within the context of predicting and preventing catastrophes, disasters, and system collapses. Mrotzek and Ossimitz (2008) acknowledged the contribution of climate change to catastrophes and employed a system's dynamic theoretical framework to model and understand common systemic structures and behaviors of catastrophes, using the Integrated Modeling Environment program at the International Institute for Applied Systems Analysis (IIASA), which served as the theoretical paradigm for the view that catastrophes comprise extreme events. Furthermore, Mrotzek and Ossimitz described several cross-disciplinary catastrophe theories including the integrated systemic theory of catastrophes (ISTC) based on Senge's general system archetypes. Their discussion on ISTC included the applicability of catastrophe archetypes, identifying and modeling of catastrophe archetypes, and finally presentation of a set of catastrophe archetypes. Mrotzek and Ossimitz concluded that the ISTC enables the identification of systemic patterns in the field of catastrophe research, informing basic patterns of modelling catastrophes. Of the six catastrophe types presented by Mrotzek and Ossimitz, overload catastrophe, overshoot catastrophe and tragedy of the commons, and creeping catastrophe might be of theoretical value to the study of organizational RRS, and consideration is given to the recommendation that catastrophe archetypes be used for inclusion of catastrophe aspects into existing models.

4.1 Organizational Collapse

Linnenluecke and Griffiths (2010) aimed at facilitating organizational development of resources and capabilities that mitigate the disastrous consequence of organizational collapse because of climate change and weather extremes using a resilience framework because an economic factor of competition approach to the former lacks the necessary tools to provide a thorough understanding. Because of the economic factors approach, past methods of coping with sudden changes have included risk and crisis adaptation mechanisms. These mechanisms were aimed at mitigating the consequences of disruptions such as strikes, changes in demand and competition, and accidents. However, the uncertainty and potentially disastrous consequences associated with climate change and extreme weather conditions are unprecedented.

4.2 Limits to Growth

Turner (2012) posed the question of whether the scenarios of the original collapse as articulated in Limits to Growth (LTG) simulation models and work of Meadows et al. (1972) were present in the events leading to the global financial crisis (GFC). In other words, if the former hypothesis is true, then the GFC could be a predictor of the collapse presented in the LTG standard run scenario. Turner (2012) thus tested his hypotheses and conducted the study using observed data over a forty-year period from 1970 to 2010 for comparative purposes to the *World3* model for three key scenarios simulated in the LTG model. Turner concluded that the observed data was in line with the standard run scenario simulated by the LTG, resulting in global collapse beginning in 2015. Furthermore, Turner's presentation and discussion of the standard run, comprehensive technology, and stabilized world scenarios from the LTG simulations shed light on the relevance of the LTG for simulation modelling work.

The observed data presented by Turner (2012) was enlightening when viewed in comparison to the graphed LTG scenarios. For population and *crude birth rates*, the observed data matched the LTG comprehensive technology scenario closely. However, the observed data for *crude death rates* followed a trajectory closer to the stabilized world scenario. In contrast, the observed data for industrial output per capita, food per capita, and services per capita were closer to the standard run scenarios, which resulted in the collapse of the LTG simulations. Finally, the author's conclusions including the fact that focus by the scientific community on climate change detracts from imminent global economic collapse; attributable to declining resources, particularly oil, is a point for further consideration.

Eastin et al. (2011) discussed the current global warming debate in relation to the LTG discourse, relating the work of Turner (2012) on Gaia to the scenarios presented in the limits to growth (LTG) model by comparing the observed data. However, in contrast to the opinion held by Turner, Eastin et al. opined that the two cases differ fundamentally, albeit share a technocratic approach to public policy. Nevertheless, Eastin et al. agreed that the standard run simulation of the LTG model is an accurate depiction of the future and clarified a key theoretical point by contrasting the problematic greater growth paradigm with the view that developing countries are the main challenge. Eastin et al. stated that this difference fundamentally narrows down to a difference in perspective (i.e., the LTG school of thought views the overarching growth paradigm as the challenge), whereas the neo-Malthusians consider the developing countries crisis to be the focus (Eastin et al.). Furthermore, sustainable development replaced the LTG paradigm in the 1980s, positing the optimistic possibility that economic growth is compatible with environmental protection and resource conservation, whereas the LTG paradigm considered growth as inimical to environmental protection (Eastin et al.).

5.0 The RRSA Management Framework for Managing Complex Problems

The purpose of the RRSA simulation study was to develop a management framework of resilience, robustness, sustainability, and adaptive capacity for organizational regimes involved in climate governance or other complex public goods games viewed as complex systems to transcend the current unsustainable state, using a quantitative computational simulation approach. The variables in the model can be extended to understand the dynamics of any complex problem such as the COVID-19 pandemic. An evolutionary game theory approach to agent-based modelling and simulation (ABMS), specifically using the prisoner's dilemma (PD) model addressed the research question of what the relationship (linear, superlinear, sublinear, power law, or other) between organizational resilience (x_1), robustness (x_2), and sustainability (x_3) and adaptive capacity (X_{t+1}) for cooperative and defective climate governance stratagems is tested and the hypothesis that a positive relationship exists between organizational resilience, robustness, and sustainability as independent variables, and the dependent variable of adaptive capacity for cooperative stratagems, else negative for defective stratagems. Greater knowledge of this relationship may be used to facilitate decision-making to move global climate change policy forward in a positive socioeconomic manner. When extended to the context of the COVID-19 pandemic, cooperative stratagems include wearing a mask, social distancing, reporting positive COVID-19 test results, self-isolating if infected, limiting travel between countries, sanitizing, and working from home. Negative stratagems include not wearing a mask, ignoring social distancing protocols, not reporting or concealing positive COVID-19 test results, not self-isolating if infected, traveling between countries without a negative COVID-19 test result, lack of sanitization, and working at the office.

An evolutionary game theory approach to agent-based modelling and simulation (ABMS), using an originally developed evolutionary prisoner's dilemma (PD) simulation on the NetLogo platform to generate the data, and statistical modelling in Excel tested the hypothesis that a positive relationship exists between resilience, robustness, and sustainability as independent variables and the dependent variable of adaptive capacity. The data generated in NetLogo was analyzed in Excel using regression analysis, with the goal of optimizing the R^2 and F-statistics while minimizing the p-values of all covariates. The null hypothesis was rejected, thus the covariates resilience, robustness, and sustainability were positively correlated with adaptive-capacity for iterated consecutive cooperative stratagems (repeated-cooperate PD) while the former covariates were negatively correlated with adaptive-capacity for iterated consecutive defective stratagems (repeated-defect PD) in the absence of an emissions penalty for climate modelling purposes.

When adapted for the purpose of understanding pandemic data, or COVID-19 data, the emissions penalty is replaced by a viral-load coefficient. The application of a viral-load coefficient to iterated consecutive defective stratagems resulted in a positive correlation between covariates and adaptive capacity. All covariates were positively correlated with adaptive capacity in run 3 of the evolutionary-RRSA PD for both cooperation and defection while for the evolutionary-tit-for-tat (TFT) PD all covariates were only positively correlated with adaptive capacity in run 3 for cooperation. In terms of game theory, several PD Nash equilibria (NE) were found. These findings were used to formulate the recommended RRSA framework discussed below.

5.1 Interpretation of Findings

Axelrod (1984) found that the tit-for-tat prisoner's dilemma (TFT PD) outperformed all other strategies for reciprocal altruism, using the scoring method for payoffs described above. While the objective of this study was not to test the efficacy of strategies for reciprocal altruism, a secondary finding, based on analysis of both payoffs and net emissions or positive COVID-19 cases as indicators of reciprocal altruism, was that the evolutionary RRSA PD outperformed all other strategies, including the evolutionary-TFT PD for reciprocal altruism. Axelrod used a *discount parameter* in his experiments, which is comparable to the emissions penalty or viral-load coefficient used in this study. Axelrod further stated that continued interaction, depending on the magnitude of his *discount parameter,* was a necessary but not sufficient condition for cooperation to emerge. The finding that the covariates' robustness and sustainability were negatively correlated with adaptive capacity in run 2 of the evolutionary-TFT PD simulation but became positively correlated with adaptive capacity in run 3 corroborates Axelrod's latter finding as run 3 included the emissions-penalty or viral-load coefficient. Both runs 2 and 3 ran for 50 timed steps, which substantiated that extended interaction is not sufficient for cooperation to emerge; however, the combination of the emissions penalty or viral-load coefficient with extended interaction in run 3 provided the necessary initial conditions for cooperation to emerge. While Axelrod's experiments on the theory of cooperation using computer-simulated PD strategies were based on game theory, he did not discuss the Nash equilibria (NE) of any of the games played in his tournaments. As NE is integral to game theory, this study expands on the work of Axelrod by including analyses of the NE for each run.

Tosun and Schoenefeld (2017) discussed that coordination of collective action into cooperation was one of the challenges of PD public goods games (PGGs), which this study both confirmed and extended upon. While defection served as a fixed-point attractor for most runs of all PD simulations except the iterated consecutive cooperation PD, application of an emissions-penalty for climate change or viral-load coefficient for COVID-19 to all strategy types (evolutionary-RRSA PD, evolutionary-TFT PD, repeated-defect PD, and repeated-cooperate PD), the latter being the exception, resulted in the coordination of collective action consisting of both cooperative and defective decision types toward increased adaptive capacity.

Hurlstone et al. (2017) further substantiated the role of collective action in successful climate negotiations for mitigating the problems of *free-riding* and *the tragedy of the commons* associated with PGGs and opined that the only PD Nash equilibrium was mutual defection known as the *paradox of cooperation* (Adami et al. 2016). Similarly, the role of collective action in the successful mitigation of COVID-19 transmission cannot be underestimated. The NE analyses for each run of the simulation indicated that mutual cooperation was a NE for the evolutionary-RRSA PD in runs 1 and 2, while defection against a cooperator and cooperation against a defector were the NEs for run 3 of the evolutionary-RRSA PD. For the evolutionary-TFT PD both mutual defection and mutual cooperation were NEs, whereas mutual cooperation was the only NE for the iterated consecutive cooperate PD, and mutual defection was the only NE for the iterated consecutive defect PD. Interpreted through the lenses of complexity theory and game theory, these findings imply that the problems of *free-riding* and the *tragedy of the commons* can be mitigated in the absence of central control, given that the parameters, which can be thought of as fostering adaptive capacity, serve as the initial conditions, which then give rise to the emergence and evolution of strategies that maximize payoffs with respect to adaptive capacity. While Adami et al. (2016), and Hurlstone et al. (2017) emphasized the importance of the coordination of collective action into cooperation, it might be too naïve and idealistic a goal as defection is inherent in all prisoner's dilemma public goods games (PD PGG) strategies and constitutes the NE for many types of PD PGGs.

The evolutionary-RRSA PD showed that the goal of steering global temperatures away from a 2°C increase by 2050 (Cole 2015), hereafter referred to as *RRSA climate negotiations,* or slowing the spread of the COVID-19 virus can be facilitated through combinations of cooperative and defective actions given the appropriate initial conditions. The primary deductions from this study was that while collective cooperation is sensitive to initial conditions, emerging and evolving were that (1) an effective framework for complex problems does not substitute top-down decision making with a polycentric bottom-up approach but rather facilitates bottom-up processes using top-down implementation with a distinction between the latter and central control; (2) defection and improved adaptive-capacity within the context of climate change and the COVID-19 pandemic are not mutually exclusive; (3) the spread of the COVID-19 virus and defection are not mutually exclusive; (4) the spread of the COVID-19 virus is sensitive to initial conditions; (5) improved resilience, robustness, sustainability and adaptive capacity to climate change or the COVID-19 virus does not necessarily involve collective coordination or control but rather emerges and evolves as a result of the initial conditions specified for the evolutionary-RRSA PD; and (6) spread of the COVID-19 virus consisting of combinations of mutual-cooperation (C, C) with defection against a cooperator (D, C), and cooperation against a defector (C, D) can lead to maximization of payoffs to self-interested parties while maintaining the goal of increasing adaptive capacity to the COVID-19 pandemic using the evolutionary-RRSA PD.

6.0 Conclusion

The perfect storm has brewed, and we find ourselves in the middle of it. Seemingly sophisticated political policies have translated unsuccessfully when implemented for the purpose of mitigating climate change, the COVID-19 pandemic and avoiding the catastrophic collapse of global systems and other malfunctions associated with capitalism. Linear feedback models do not adequately capture the dynamics of complex systems. The RRSA management model is a computational simulation tool for managing complex global problems. A shift away from the current global crisis calls for shifts in thinking away from shallowness, self-change, lowering consumption through innovation, technological advancement, and longer planning horizons. This type of personal and global systemic real growth will take decades to achieve without a universal intervention, which is when nature intervenes, takes the reins and massive change is catalyzed through global warming, climate change, and epidemic or pandemic events. The significant and far-reaching implication for applied change management is that organizations should be viewed as systems capable of self-organization in the sense that effective processes, structures, and strategies emerge and evolve from teleological bottom-up processes comparative to biological self-organizing systems, informing the role of managers and leaders in the creation of agile, resilient, robust, sustainable organizations capable of achieving adaptive capacity to global catastrophic collapse.

References

Adami, C., Schossau, J., and Hintze, M. 2016. "Models of evolution and evolutionary game theory: A comment on 'evolutionary game theory using agent-based models.'" *Physics of Life Reviews,* 19, 32–35. https://doi.org/10.1016/j.plrev.2016.11.003.

Amemiya-Ramírez, M. 2014. "Sustainable technology assessment and sustainable scenarios of techno social phenomena." *Journal of Sociocybernetics,* 12 (1/2): 53-65. https://doi.org/10.26754/ojs_jos/jos.20141/2794.

Anderies, J. M., C. Folke, B. Walker, and E. Ostrom. 2013. "Aligning key concepts for global change policy: robustness, resilience, and sustainability." *Ecology and Society* 18 (2): 8. https://doi.org/10.5751/ES-05178-180208.

Ansell, C., and Gash, A. (2008). "Collaborative governance in theory and practice." *Journal of Public Administration Research and Theory,* 18 (4): 543–571. https://doi.org/10.1093/jopart/mum032.

Axelrod, R. 1984. *The Evolution of Cooperation.* Basic Books.

Ay, N., Der, R. and Prokopenko, M. (2012) Guided self-organization: Perception–action loops of embodied systems. *Theory in Biosciences.* 131, 125–127. https://doi.org/10.1007/s12064-011-0140-1.

Bahadur, A. V., Ibrahim, M., and Tanner, T. 2010. "The resilience renaissance? Unpacking of resilience for tackling climate change and disasters." *Institute of Development Studies.* http://dev2.opendocs.ids.ac.uk/opendocs/bitstream/handle/123456789/2368/The%20resilience%20renaissance.pdf?sequence=1.

Elkington, J. 1994. "Towards the sustainable corporation: Win-win-win business strategies for sustainable development."

California Management Review, *36*(2), 90–100. https://doi. org/10.2307/41165746.

Eastin, J., Grundmann, R., and Prakash, A. 2011. "The two limits debates: 'Limits to growth' and climate change." *Futures,* 43 (1): 16–26. https://doi.org/10.1016/j.futures.2010.03.001.

Engle, N. L. 2011. "Adaptive capacity and its assessment." *Global Environmental Change,* 21 (2): 647–656. https://doi.org/10.1016/j. gloenvcha.2011.01.019.

Fiksel, J. 2006. "Sustainability and resilience: toward a systems approach." *Sustainability: Science Practice and Policy,* *2*(2), 14–21. Retrieved from http://geminis.dma.ulpgc.es/profesores/personal/ jmpc/Master08(SegundaEdici%F3n)/PARA%20EL%20 MASTER%20SEGUNDA%20EDICION/Fiksel.pdf.

Fiksel, J., Bruins, R., Gatchett, A., Gilliland, A., and Brink, M. 2014. "The triple value model: a systems approach to sustainable solutions." *Clean Technologies and Environmental Policy,* 16 (4): 691–702. https://doi.org/10.1007/s10098-013-0696-1.

Folke, C. 2006. "Resilience: The emergence of a perspective for social–ecological systems analyses." *Global Environmental Change,* 16 (3): 253–267. https://doi.org/10.1016/j.gloenvcha.2006.04.002.

Folke, C., Hahn, T., Olsson, P., and Norberg, J. 2005. "Adaptive governance of social-ecological systems." *Annual Review of Environment and Resources,* *30,* 441–473. https://doi.org/10.1146/ annurev.energy.30.050504.144511.

Gershenson, C. 2011. "Complexity at large." *Complexity,* 17 (1): 1–4. https://doi.org/10.1002/cplx.20383.

Götz, G., and Schäffler, A. 2015. "Conundrums in implementing a green economy in the Gauteng City-Region." *Current Opinion in*

Environmental Sustainability, 13, 79–87. https://doi.org/10.1016/j. cosust.2015.02.005.

Holling, C. S. 1973. "Resilience and stability of ecological systems." *Annual Review of Ecology and Systematics, 4,* 1–23. https://www. jstor.org/stable/2096802.

Hurlstone, M. J., Wang, S., Price, A., Leviston, Z., and Walker, I. 2017. "Cooperation studies of catastrophe avoidance: implications for climate negotiations." *Climatic Change,* 1–15. https://doi. org/10.1007/s10584-016-1838-3.

International Organization for Standardization. 2015. "ISO 26000 and the international integrated reporting <IR> framework briefing summary." ISO.org. https://www.iso.org/files/live/sites/isoorg/ files/store/en/PUB100402.pdf.

Kuecker, G. 2007. "The perfect storm: Catastrophic collapse in the 21st century." *The International Journal of Environmental, Cultural, Economic, and Social Sustainability,* 3 (5), 1–10. https://ijs. cgpublisher.com/product/pub.41/prod.350.

Kuecker, G. 2020. "The Perfect Storm's Pandemic-driven Soft Collapse." *The International Journal of Environmental, Cultural, Economic, and Social Sustainability: Annual Review 16* (1): 1–18. https://doi. org/10.18848/1832-2077/CGP/v16i01/1-18.

Lemos, M. C., Agrawal, A., Eakin, H., Nelson, D. R., Engle, N. L., and Johns, O. 2013. "Building adaptive capacity to climate change in less developed countries." In *Climate Science for Serving Society,* edited by G. Asrar and J. Hurrell, 437–457. Springer. https://doi. org/10.1007/978-94-007-6692-1_16.

Linnenluecke, M., and Griffiths, A. 2010. "Beyond adaptation: resilience for business in light of climate change and weather extremes." *Business and Society.* https://doi.org/10.1177/0007650310368814

Munang, R., Thiaw, I., Alverson, K., Liu, J., and Han, Z. 2013. "The role of ecosystem services in climate change adaptation and disaster risk reduction." *Current Opinion in Environmental Sustainability*, 5 (1): 47–52. doi:10.1016/j.cosust.2013.02.002.

Mayunga, J. S. 2007. "Understanding and applying the concept of community disaster resilience: A capital-based approach." *Summer academy for social vulnerability and resilience building*, 1, 16. https://www.u-cursos.cl/usuario/3b514b53bcb4025aaf9a6781047e4a66/mi_blog/r/11._Joseph_S._Mayunga.pdf.

McEvoy, D., Fünfgeld, H., and Bosomworth, K. 2013. "Resilience and climate change adaptation: The importance of framing." *Planning Practice and Research*, 28 (3): 1–14. https://doi.org/10.1080/02697459.2013.787710.

Motesharrei, S., Rivas, J., and Kalnay, E. 2014. "Human and Nature Dynamics (HANDY): Modeling inequality and use of resources in the collapse or sustainability of societies." *Ecological Economics*, 101, 90–102. https://doi.org/10.1016/j.ecolecon.2014.02.0140418.

Mrotzek, M., and Ossimitz, G. 2008. "Catastrophe archetypes-using system dynamics to build an integrated systemic theory of catastrophes." *IDIMT-2008-Managing the Unmanageable-16th Interdisciplinary Information Management Talks*, 3671-384. https://pdfs.semanticscholar.org/5977/11a7e3f56af745f8982894bd684422381e3c.pdf.

Munang, R., Thiaw, I., Alverson, K., Liu, J., and Han, Z. 2013. "The role of ecosystem services in climate change adaptation and disaster risk reduction." *Current Opinion in Environmental Sustainability*, 5 (1): 47–52. https://doi.org/10.1016/j.cosust.2013.02.002.

Nelson, D. R., Adger, W. N., and Brown, K. 2007. "Adaptation to environmental change: contributions of a resilience framework."

Annual Review of Environment and Resources, 32 (1): 395. https://doi.org/10.1146/annurev.energy.32.051807.090348.

Oliver, T. H., Heard, M. S., Isaac, N. J. B., Roy, D. B., Procter, D., Eigenbrod, F., Freckleton, R., Hector, A., Orme, C. D. L., Petchey, O. L., Proenca, V., Raffaelli, D., Suttle, K. B., Mace, G. M., Martin-Lopez, B., Woodcock, B. A., and Bullock, J. M. 2015. "Biodiversity and resilience of ecosystem functions." *Trends in Ecology & Evolution*, 30 (11): 673–684. https://doi.org/10.1016/j.tree.2015.08.009.

Polani, D., Prokopenko, M., and Yaeger, L. S. 2013. "Information and self-organization of behavior." *Advances in Complex Systems*, 16 (02n03). https://doi.org/10.1142/S021952591303001X.

Ram, K. 2017. *A Complex Systems Simulation Study for Increasing Adaptive-Capacity* (Doctoral dissertation, Walden University). ProQuest Dissertations Publishing. https://www.proquest.com/openview/0dc19cf89f78b76cfeb4f1c64b8b1b69/1?pq-origsite=gscholar&cbl=18750.

Ram, K. 2018. "Complexity: The tipping point for leadership." In B. S. Thakkar (Ed.), *The Future of Leadership*, 93–124. Palgrave Macmillan.

Reeves, M., and Deimler, M. 2011. "Adaptability: The new competitive advantage." *Harvard Business Review*, 135–41. doi:10.1002/9781119204084.ch2.

Slaper, T. F., and Hall, T. J. 2011. "The triple bottom line: what is it and how does it work." *Indiana Business Review*, 86 (1): 4–8. http://www.ibrc.indiana.edu/ibr/2011/spring/article2.html.

Solow, R. M. 1957. "Technical change and the aggregate production function." *The Review of Economics and Statistics*, 39 (3): 312–320. MIT Press. http://www.jstor.org/stable/1926047?origin=JSTOR-pdf.

Tosun, J., and Schoenefeld, J. J. 2017. "Collective climate action and networked climate governance." *Wiley Interdisciplinary Reviews: Climate Change,* 8 (1). https://doi.org/10.1002/wcc.440.

Turner, G. M. 2012. "On the cusp of global collapse? Updated comparison of The Limits to Growth with historical data." *GAIA-Ecological Perspectives for Science and Society,* 21 (2): 116–124. http://www.ingentaconnect.com/content/oekom/gaia/2012/00000021/00000002/art00010?crawler=true.

Watts, D. 2014. *Six Degrees: The New Science of Networks.* Random House.

Whitacre, J., and Bender, A. 2010. "Degeneracy: a design principle for achieving robustness and evolvability." *Journal of Theoretical Biology, 263*(1), 143–153. https://doi.org/10.1016/j.jtbi.2009.11.008.

CHAPTER 2

Business and Social Challenges from Unexpected Global Events

by Kevin M. Sorbello

Abstract

The potential business and social impact of unexpected global events were painfully evident during the COVID-19 pandemic, changing what was previously considered normal societal activity and work environments into what many are calling the *new normal*. From where people work or study, how they greet one another to how they enter the workplace, stores, or sports events, life may never be the same. With these potential changes in mind, are governmental and business leaders and managers acting appropriately or overreacting? There have certainly been greater pandemics as far as lethality, so why are societies so ready to change based on a virus that showed less than 1% crude mortality rate for the general population? Whether these changes are due to social awareness, medical opinion, political opportunism, or fear generated by poorly informed or misinformed news and social media outlets, they create leadership and management challenges on a global scale. Will the new model of business and social norms shift back over time once more information on the details surrounding the spread and lethality of the pandemic come to light, or do recent reactions signal an ever-changing landscape? Humans are social animals and guidelines on how they must stay distant from one another, wear masks, sanitize, and avoid physical contact may have lasting effects on their mental health and how they treat one another. What will the future landscape of work, school, shopping, and social gatherings look like? How engrained or changeable are previous social norms? Workers will look to their managers and leaders for guidance in this new and uncertain landscape, and short of complete, factual information, decisions on how to proceed and protect the workforce while continuing to remain productive and profitable will weigh heavily on their shoulders. The COVID-19 pandemic may be the poster child for unexpected global events yet provides a historic point from which businesses and governments will need to plan for reactions that affect society and businesses on a global scale. This chapter will explore these issues using current knowledge of policy and projections by social, business, and health experts on what changes and challenges lie ahead for change managers in the current and post-pandemic world.

Keywords: COVID, pandemic, new normal, supply chains, global events

1. What Just Happened?

If you're not confused, you're not paying attention.
—Tom Peters, *Thriving on Chaos: Handbook for a Management Revolution*

January 9, 2020: The World Health Organization (WHO) publicly announced fifty-nine cases of a new COVID virus discovered in Wuhan, China (*American Journal of Managed Care* [*AJMC*], 2021). The virus, similar to pneumonia cases, emerged in Wuhan City in December 2019. The studies revealed that it was a new, or novel, form of the coronavirus not previously described (Atalan 2020). The virus was therefore called coronavirus 2019, abbreviated as COVID-19 (AJMC 2021). Coronaviruses exist in seven known forms; four are common influenza pathogens known as variations of the common cold; one is MERS-CoV, and the other two are SARS-CoV. Of these seven, MERS-CoV and SARS-CoV2 (COVID-19) are severe respiratory illnesses although SARS-CoV1 has a higher mortality rate (Baba et al. 2021).

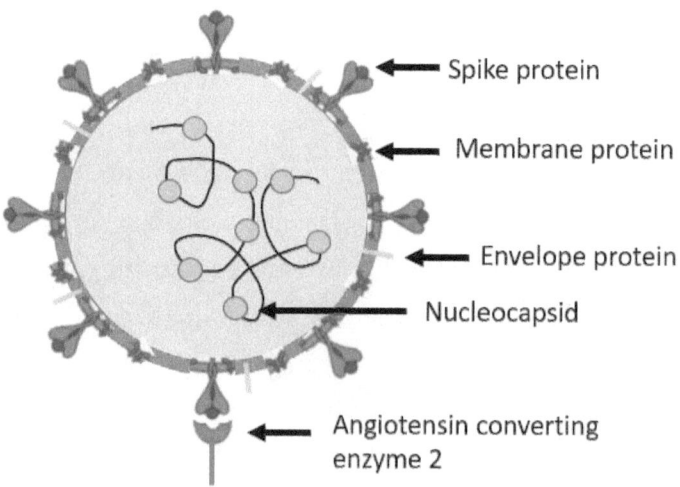

Figure 1. The Structure of the COVID-19 Virus

Note: The nucleocapsid forms complexes with the virus's genomic RNA and interacts with the membrane proteins during virion assembly.

January 20, 2020: The US Center for Disease Control (CDC) began screening passengers at JFK International, San Francisco

International, and Los Angeles International airports. These airports were targeted because they represented the greatest number of incoming passengers from Wuhan. The next day, January 21, the CDC confirmed the first US case of COVID-19 in a Washington State resident who had returned from Wuhan on January 15, 2020. Two days later, on January 23, Wuhan went under quarantine with 13 deaths and an additional 300 sickened with the virus. China not only closed of Wuhan's 11 million population but restricted access to Huanggang, resulting in a lockdown of up to 18 million Chinese citizens. The WHO issued a global health emergency on January 31 as the death toll climbed to 200 with another 9,800 confirmed cases. They noted these cases were distributed between the US, Germany, Japan, Vietnam, China, and Taiwan.

February 3, 2020: The reaction in the US escalated with a declaration by then Pres. Donald Trump of a US public health emergency. By February 25, 2020, the CDC indicated COVID-19 met two of the three requirements for a pandemic with the third criteria of a worldwide spread not yet detected. By March 6, 21 out of 3,500 passengers on a California cruise ship had tested positive for the virus, resulting in the ship being put into quarantine at sea rather than being allowed to dock in San Francisco. Sixty passengers on that ship would later sue Carnival Corp for gross negligence in how their safety was handled.

March 11, 2020: A quick escalation around the world as the CDC finally declared COVID-19 as a pandemic.

March 13, 2020: President Trump declares COVID-19 a national emergency with travel bans on non-US citizens traveling from 26 European countries.

March 17, 2020: The University of Minnesota begins testing hydroxychloroquine treatment on 1,500 people at high risk of exposure to see if it could prevent those exposed to the virus from becoming sick or at least reduce the severity of the infection. President Trump asks Congress to expedite emergency relief checks to Americans as the US death toll rose to 100.

March 19, 2020: California governor issues a stay-at-home order for all residents except to go to an essential job or shop for essentials while instructing health care centers to prioritize service to those exhibiting the most severe symptoms. Mandate results in restricted access to hospitals quickly overwhelmed by unprecedented admissions of COVID-19 patients.

March 24, 2020: Focus on patient treatment results in a delay of new clinical trials. Center for Biosimilar reports drugs with FDA approval are unlikely to make it into circulation while hospitals are struggling to find enough personal protective equipment. Although the CDC and medical professionals had warned for decades of the possibility of a global pandemic, and despite knowing the chances the pandemic would be a variant of SARS, affecting the respiratory system and potentially transmittable by air, no provisions had been made to increase the supply of protective equipment or respirators. This failure to prepare, even when such a situation was predicted by health care workers well in advance (Jiang et al. 2020), exemplifies the need for businesses to prepare for potential global events rather than scramble and place blame once the predictable event occurs. There is little excuse for the lack of preparation and the resulting finger-pointing noted during the pandemic. States that looked to the federal government for aid and blamed legislative and executive branches for not providing such equipment ignore the responsibility of those who had the knowledge, finances, and time to better prepare for a situation identified by their own experts long in advance.

March 25, 2020: CARES Act, an FDA emergency use authorization to use hydroxychloroquine, is passed by U.S. Congress and signed into law on March 27. A study report in JAMA Ophthalmology revealed 38 patients from Hubei Province, China, had contracted COVID-19 through the eye, contradicting transmission assumptions made by other leading professional societies. Health agencies working on the pandemic were focused on patient care and potential vaccine contracts during April and May 2020 while the US death toll from COVID-19 passes the 100,000 mark.

June 10, 2020: The number of confirmed cases reaches two million. However, some question the number of deaths attributed to COVID-19 with speculation that the numbers are possibly being inflated by certain sectors trying to capitalize on government funding provided to hospitals based on COVID-19 responsible deaths.

June 16, 2020: US officials working on *Operation Warp Speed*, a project to rapidly develop and deploy a COVID-19 vaccine, indicate they would make vaccines available at no cost to elderly patients once released under FDA emergency use authority.

June 18, 2020: The World Health Organization (WHO) announces it will stop testing hydroxychloroquine as a treatment; two days later the National Institutes of Health (NIH) halts its trials of the drug, indicating treatment does no harm while offering no benefit.

June 22, 2020: A study published in *Science Translational Medicine* suggests up to 80% of Americans who sought treatment for flu-like symptoms were actually infected with COVID-19, amounting to around 8.7 million US infections.

June 30, 2020: White House medical representative Dr. Fauci, a respected virologist, warns new cases could rise to 100,000 per day based on the measured trajectory of infections.

July 2020: U.S. states reverse reopening plans and scientists call on the WHO to revise COVID-19 precautions based on the potential for the virus to be an airborne virus, not just a virus spread by small droplets from the nose or mouth. Dr. Fauci, who had originally gone on record on the lack of protection offered by wearing masks, reverses his position on masks and issues strong statements in support of wearing them in public. The apparent reversal of the WHO position in regard to cause, effects, response, and source of the virus, results in the US beginning its withdrawal from the WHO due to a lack of confidence. President Trump notifies the United Nations of the decision, which would not take effect until 2021, that the decision to withdraw could be reversed by incoming President Biden. With the daily infection rates rising to 75,600, hospitals indicate they are unable to address other critical diseases such as cancer. A report in *The Lancet Oncology* suggests that delays in cancer diagnosis, referrals, and treatment could result in almost 10% more deaths in England over the following 5 years.

The immediacy of the need to find a vaccine results in massive funding for research. The US agrees to a $2.1 billion deal with GlaxoSmithKline and Sanofi Pasteur to develop, manufacture, and deliver a vaccine. Another $1.5 billion deal is made with Moderna for 100 million doses of its mRNA-1273 vaccine even while the vaccine is still conducting phase 3 trials with the National Institute of Allergy and Infectious Diseases and the Biomedical Advanced Research and Development Authority (AJMC 2021).

September 8, 2020: AstraZeneca halts their phase 3 trials to conduct a safety data review following an unknown adverse reaction in a UK patient. Pfizer and BioNTech announce an expansion of their phase 3 trials from 30,000 to 40,000 to include tests on patients as young as 16 years and patients with HIV and hepatitis B or C.

December 2020: COVID-19 delta variant is identified in India and believed to be more than twice as contagious as previous variants and more likely to result in hospitalizations. The CDC labels the delta strain as a variant of concern (VOC). As of November 19, 2021, this variant represents more than 99% of all COVID-19 infections (Katella 2021).

November 26, 2021: World Health Organization (WHO) designates a new variant, omicron (B.1.1.529) as a VOC. The decision was based on the fact omicron has several mutations that have an impact on how it spreads and its severity, especially since some cases are extremely mild while others require hospitalization (WHO 2021).

2. Who Names the Variants and What Does It All Mean?

The U.S. Department of Health and Human Services (HHS) established a SARS-CoV-2 Interagency Group called the SIG. The group was designed to enhance coordination among CDC, NIH, FDA, BARDA, and DoD (CDC, 2021). The SIG meets regularly to evaluate variant risks, potential countermeasures, vaccines, therapeutics, and diagnostics. The variants are put into five potential categories: Variants being monitored (VBM); Variant of Interest (VOI); Variant of Concern (VOC); Variant Under Monitoring (VUM), and Variant of High Consequence (VOHC) (WHO, 2021). There are two names or designations given to each variant. The Pango Lineage is a scientific designator that could be confusing to the general public, so the World Health Organization (WHO) gives each variant a Greek letter label. The first variant from the original virus, known as the novel corona virus, was the Alpha variant, considered a VOC on December 29, 2020, then designated a VBM by September 21, 2021. The next two variants, Beta and Gamma, received the same VOC and VBM designations on the same dates as the Alpha variant. However, the Epsilon variant designated as a VOC on March 19, 2021, was upgraded to a VOI twice; first on February 26, 2021, then again on June 29, 2021 due to minor changes noted in the Pango Lineage. The next five variants were labeled Eta, Iota, Kappa, Zeta, and Mu, which were designated as VOI and VBM by September 21, 2021. Of all the variants, only five have been designated as VOCs: Alpha, Beta, Gamma, Delta, and Omicron. The Delta variant was first identified in India, with the Omicron starting in South Africa, but quickly identified in multiple countries by November of 2021. The difference between the Delta and Omicron variants can best be described by differences in mortality and communicability. The Delta variant poses a greater risk of hospitalization and death and was noted as being 60% more transmissible than the Alpha variant, while the Omicron is less severe, but has a much higher transmissibility than the Delta variant and may help the virus partially evade the vaccines (LiveScience, 2021).

3. What Follows?

The following months prior to the release of three vaccine options by Pfizer, Moderna, and Johnson & Johnson pharmaceuticals bore witness to political infighting, finger-pointing, revisionist history, and continued changes in recommendations on how to prevent the spread of the virus and whether it was airborne. Initial instructions to wipe down packages with disinfectants (alcohol), wait times between deliveries and opening of packages, social distancing inside and outside buildings, and other guidance were routinely revised or discarded as more information was obtained through the study. An example of these reversals can be seen in the August 25 CDC reversal on the decision not to test asymptomatic people who had been exposed when it was revealed the decision had bypassed the CDC's usual scientific review process and lacked internal review. A day later the FDC grants emergency use authorization for the Abbott's Rapid Test, a portable COVID-19 test. Another example is the September 21 reversal of CDC's previous claim the virus was airborne. This reversal came on the same day Johnson & Johnson began their own phase 3 trials in 60,000 patients with a single shot vaccine that did not require freezing the vaccine between production and use. The push for a viable vaccine continued as the number of worldwide deaths reportedly due to COVID-19 exceeded 1 million. The outgoing Trump administration signed a $486 million agreement on October 9 with AstraZeneca to produce its AZD7442 cocktail of two monoclonal antibodies. About the same time, Johnson & Johnson halted recruitment for its phase 3 trials when *POLITICO* reported an unexplained illness, then quickly returned to testing on October 23 indicating such halts were common during phase 3 trials. By the end of 2020, three viable vaccines were authorized for emergency use by the FDA: Pfizer, Moderna, and Johnson & Johnson while the UK authorized AstraZeneca and Oxford COVID-19 vaccines.

4. In Whom Do We Trust?

> It's funny. All you have to do is say something nobody understands and they'll do practically anything you want them to.
> —J. D. Salinger, *The Catcher in the Rye*

Although governments indicated they would follow the science of the virus, their actions and policies were and are often in opposition to the science. US House Speaker Pelosi mandated the wearing of masks while in session even by those who had been vaccinated yet routinely met outside such sessions without a mask and near others even though the CDC indicated such a policy for those already vaccinated was unnecessary. Other politicians at the state level, such as California governor Gavin Newsom, mandated the wearing of masks and the closing of businesses yet routinely went to restaurants without a mask and held parties where the participants were near one another. Meanwhile, news media outlets were polarized in their coverage of these issues with some ignoring the paradoxes and hypocrisy while others spent an inordinate amount of time covering them. The virus and how people should react to it became a political weapon by the ruling party, and the control they had over social media became obvious during attempts to restrict or deny access to those media outlets by those who opposed the position or doubted the information being presented. Former President Trump, for example, was banned from Facebook, Twitter, and other social media platforms while foreign dictators and terror organizations were allowed to post misinformation and anti-American propaganda without censure.

The difficulty in predicting how a pandemic will unfold outside of the medical aspects led to reactions that erred on the extreme side of caution. Lockdowns and quarantines of businesses were conducted on a worldwide basis (Atalan 2020). Schools were closed although studies showed children would neither catch nor transmit the virus and when reopened were required to wear masks disregarding other studies suggesting adverse effects due to increased CO_2 levels of children wearing masks. An estimated 1.725 billion students worldwide were affected by school closures in April 2020 (Masoud and Bohra 2020). The psychological impact of social isolation resulting from long-term lockdowns has led mental health professionals to believe the world may face a parallel pandemic of acute stress disorders, posttraumatic stress disorders, emotional disturbance, sleep disorders, depressive syndromes, and potential suicides (Mucci et al. 2020). The psychological damage from children being isolated during their formative years may take decades to discover while the suicides rates dramatically increased in response to school closures. Teachers' unions refused to return teachers to classrooms until they received vaccinations while some who had been vaccinated still refused to return. Meanwhile, teachers who refused to hold in-class education for children who were U.S. citizens held in-class education for illegal immigrants who had been allowed to enter the country without COVID-19 vaccination even though a significant number of these immigrants had tested positive for COVID-19. Parents of U.S. students were justifiably angered at the apparent hypocrisy demonstrated by the educational system, particularly the teachers' unions that ignored the science they touted.

The reaction of U.S. governors was also varied. Some states enacted strict stay-at-home orders, mask mandates, and restaurant and school closures while other states took lesser measures. The results of these opposite approaches have caused great debates on how the numbers are being used by proponents and opponents of each methodology (King et al. 2021). Some argued that non-lockdown states had 75% fewer COVID-19-related per-capita fatalities in more rural states (*The Editorial Board*, 2020; Yang 2020). The differences between Florida, New York, and California's approaches to the pandemic were dramatic with California and New York imposing the toughest measures. However, analysis of collected data suggests Florida's less aggressive measures resulted in fewer hospitalizations and deaths despite having a larger senior population (King et al. 2021; Njolomole 2020). While those supporting less drastic measures point to the success of Florida Governor DeSantis's approach, others claim the data is flawed due to underreporting of cases (*The Poynter Institute*, 2021). Businesses were frustrated with differences in restrictions that appeared contrary to the data being to state officials who controlled not only how they could operate but whether they could operate at all.

The general population was likewise frustrated on several fronts. While teachers stayed home and taught in virtual classrooms, police, fire departments, grocery store workers, and those who supplied them went to work and interacted with populations that were likely exposed to or had already contracted the virus. Many businesses closed due to state stay-home mandates, and when those mandates were lifted, they were unable to attract workers back to the workplace due to the government providing funds to unemployed workers at a level that exceeded their previous take-home salary. Other businesses were frustrated because government funds were provided to minority businesses, excluding those operated by white business owners. The inequity of support by a government who advocated equity further divided the population. The shift in political power that occurred during the pandemic was due in large part to emergency voting efforts put in place that were ostensibly designed to allow greater voter turnout during a time of restricted access. These policies, however, allowed voter irregularities that might have affected the outcome of the election, and although initially meant as a temporary way to address access for an election, it represented initiatives that had been presented and denied for years and once approved were touted as a permanent change to election rules. States that reacted to these potential changes by requiring voter identification in the form of a driver's license, government-issued identification, or the last four digits of the voter's social security number were called racist and a new form of racial discrimination exceeding such discrimination banned decades before. The hyperbole from all levels of government further confused and polarized the public who increasingly showed their distrust of the media and government in general.

5. Figures Lie and Liars Figure

The current US Government's representatives indicated they wanted to follow the science. The reality, however, was that they did not follow the science nor did the scientific representatives follow their own guidance. McNulty (2021) argued the use of PCR testing (polymerase chain reaction) should not be used as an indicator of an epidemic, primarily since it is a qualitative result merely indicating the presence of the virus, not a quantitative one. In other words, simple detection of viral RNA does not necessarily indicate the presence of an infectious virus or a causative agent for clinical symptoms. PCR tests magnify DNA samples and the magnification is measured by the number of cycles needed to make the target DNA visible. This is known as the Cycle Threshold (Ct) or Quantification Cycle (Cq) number, where the higher the number of cycles represent the lower amount of DNA in the test sample. The result is that these tests can magnify a small sample of DNA, whether it is from a dead or active virus, millions of times. PCR testing is used to magnify DNA samples for the purpose of identifying trace DNA in crime scenes, yet the presence of DNA does not in and of itself certify the suspect or the cause of death; it merely indicates some trace amount of the DNA was present.

The qualitative nature of PCR testing may be one of the underlying reasons why there are no international standards for PCR tests, particularly since the results can vary by a million times, from country to country and from test to test. PCR testing for the presence of COVID-19 in a patient admitted for symptoms does not, therefore, mean they are suffering from COVID-19, it only means they have some amount of the virus present in their system.

The question then becomes, "What about all those who have died from COVID-19?" To answer that question a person would have to know whether a COVID-19 "related" illness was responsible, or COVID was the true cause of death. The reported death increase due to COVID-19 was in opposition to the noted decrease in Flu related deaths, even though both exhibit similar symptoms. Perhaps a look at the national death rate for the US between 2019 and 2021 might show a significant increase based on the more than 450,000 reported COVID-19 deaths during that period.

This is where things get a little confusing and complicated. Figure 2 represents the deaths per 1000 in the US between 2019 and 2021. Based on this data, one might assume the increase in deaths are dramatic and obviously due to the COVID-19 pandemic.

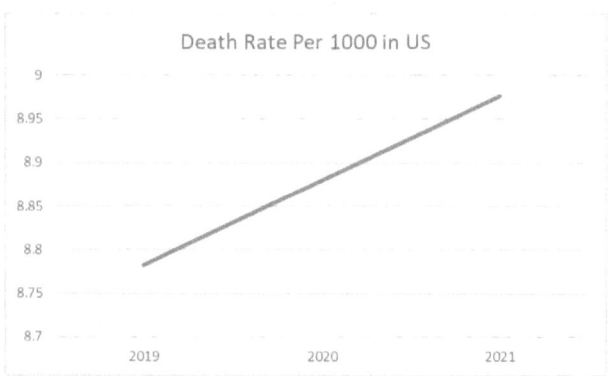

Figure 2. Deaths per 1000 in the US 2019-2021

Note: CDC-based data obtained from macrotrends.net

Figure 2 is a good example of how data can be manipulated to prove a point made by someone with an agenda. Why? Because it lacks historical context. Figure 2 provides a little more context by showing the death rate per 1000 in the US between 2013 and 2021.

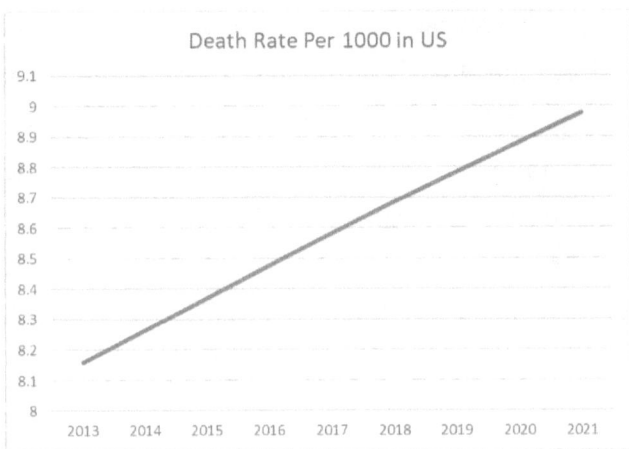

Figure 3. Deaths per 1000 in the US 2013-2021

Note: CDC-based data obtained from macrotrends.net

Figure 3 shows that the apparently high increase in the death rate per 1000 actually started in 2013, at least six years before the appearance of COVID-19. The problem with Figure 2 is that it would not support the idea that COVID-19 significantly increased the national death rate. Figure 4 adds a little more context to how the death rate per 1000 has changed by going back to the year 2000.

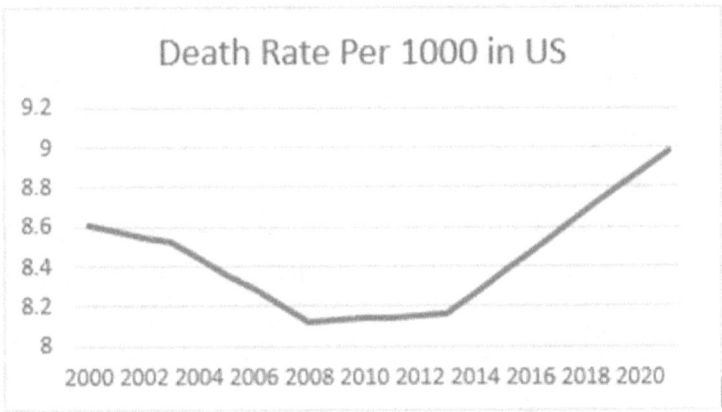

Figure 4. Deaths per 1000 in the US 2000-2021

Note: CDC-based data obtained from macrotrends.net

Figure 4 shows that the death rate per 1000 had a marked shift downwards from 2000 to 2008, followed by a minor increase until 2013, after which it increased dramatically. "Dramatically," however, is a deceptive term. A close look at the vertical axis shows that the data actually varies from a low near 8.1 to a high of 8.9 between 2000 and 2021. This represents less than a change of 1 person per 1000. To get a better feel for how the death rate has changed since 2000, Figure 5 shows the same data based on a 0 to 10 deaths by 1000 scale.

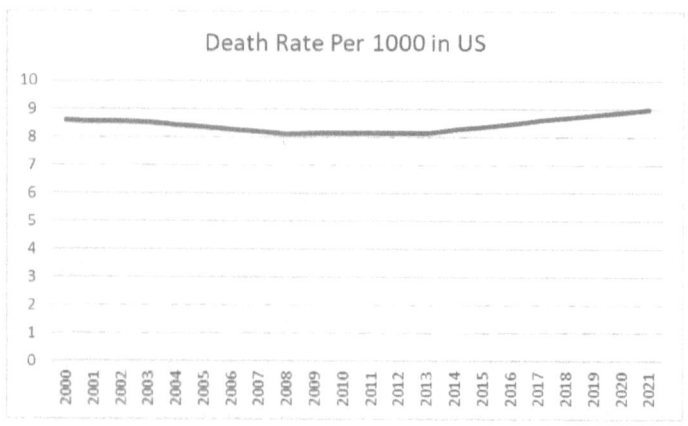

Figure 5. Deaths per 1000 in the US 2000-2021 (0 – 10 scale)

Note: CDC-based data obtained from macrotrends.net

Figure 5 shows a fluctuation of less than a one death per 1000 over a 21-year span. This figure would not support someone whose intention was to show a significant increase in the death rate between 2019 and 2020, yet Figure 1, based on the same data, would suggest COVID-19 was responsible for a significant increase in US deaths during that period.

These examples show how easily data or "facts" can be distorted in their presentation or telling. It also would indicate there was no significant increase in the death rate due to COVID-19. Fluctuations in the death rate up to 1 per 1000 represents a variation in total deaths of up to 348,000 based on a US population of 348,000,000; a figure that represents approximately 78% of the reported 448,000 deaths attributed to COVID-19. However, the remaining deaths could represent an increased number of deaths due to causes other than COVID-19, such as suicide and other illnesses that were left untreated due to hospitals prioritizing COVID-19 patients over others with serious illnesses.

McNulty's (2021) warning about the use of PCR testing takes on a greater importance after reviewing the data related to deaths per 1000 since 2013. His quoting of Paracelsus's 1538 argument that "all things are poison, and nothing is without poison; the dosage alone makes the poison," a possible source for the adage "dosis sola facit venunum" (the dose alone makes the poison), warns against using any evidence of a virus as a reason to blame the virus for all virus-like symptoms. The minimum infection dose (MID) for major respiratory and enteric viruses, including COVID, is estimated at around 100 particles. This, however, is not the threshold used for determining COVID related deaths; PCR testing has become the significant indicator, even though never intended to be used in that manner.

Other virus outbreaks that were touted as pandemics, such as the whooping cough in New Hampshire and the Swine Flu panic of 2009, turned out to be false alarms. The difference between how the media treated those false alarms and the COVID-19 "pandemic" has more to do with politics, political agendas, the need for the media to promote their programs to increase revenue, and in some cases, to support the agendas of the political groups and agendas they support. The media's doomsday predications and distortion of the facts led to a significant effort to produce a vaccine under emergency protocols. While the need to produce a vaccine was an important step, conflicting and often contradictory mandates and warnings confused the public and allowed new measures to be put in place that arguably benefitted one political party over the other. The biggest problem, however, was the creation of a never-ending string of mandates and fear mongering based on new variants of the virus before the dangers of the new variants were fully understood. The use, therefore, of distorted reporting and non-contextual data presentations has created an atmosphere of doubt and served to split society into factions that either accept the changes that decrease personal freedom and those who resist mandates and the draconian measures introduced to promote specific political agendas. The lack of unbiased media coverage further exacerbates the confusion and distrust, to varying degrees, around the world.

6. Side Effects and Social Unrest

Several social, psychological, and economic reactions and side effects of the pandemic were unexpected, such as a call in the US to defund the police led by leftist extremists who believed the police were the root cause of crime against minorities. While statistics showed, for example, that a white suspect was more likely to be shot by the police than a black suspect (Johnson et al. 2019; Mac Donald 2020), violent protests were formed in response to a few black deaths at the hands of white police officers. Ignored were the hundreds of deaths of minorities caused by minorities in a single week by those whose agenda was to create social unrest to which their political party could use as capital toward the next election cycle. The result of these efforts was the actual defunding and demonizing of police officers, which in turn resulted in increased rates of retirements or resignations. The impact of these reductions was exacerbated by laws that allowed suspects, even those accused of murder, to be released without bail, where many committed additional crimes once released. Other changes resulted in changing the focus of law enforcement to more violent crimes, allowing shoplifting to go unpunished if the total cost of the items was less than $900. Shoplifting rose to such a level that some stores closed outlets, others reduced operating hours, and others simply passed on their losses to law-abiding customers who watched as shoplifters simply walked out of the store with backpacks full of stolen merchandise. One shopping clerk was killed while attempting to stop a shoplifter, and the suspect was never captured. Police were also hesitant to confront suspects who belonged to a minority, especially black suspects since such apprehensions were commonly recorded by citizens in proximity. Such interactions could result in jail time, death threats, and loss of employment for police officers. Many police officers decided it was safer to allow a suspect to go free than risk punishment for doing their job. The result in some cities was complete chaos with cities such as Portland, Oregon, seeing riots, looting, and buildings burned for months. Meanwhile, some politicians were noted as justifying looting as being a way to compensate those who had been oppressed by a society built by and operated by systemic white supremacy. The rhetoric spewed by a vocal minority, supported by progressive media and extreme political ideology by those in power at that time, created further social divisions and problems for businesses.

Another side effect of the pandemic was a change to election laws that may have altered the outcome of the 2020 elections. Some argued that this change, allowing ballot harvesting and undocumented voting, resulted in a different election outcome than predicted. The end result was the election of government representatives that shifted away from energy independence by shutting down and attempting to shut down fossil fuel pipelines and production in favor of creating a solar- and wind-powered energy system. Meanwhile, these same officials approved of a similar pipeline that would support Russian interests and potentially harm Ukraine, something former President Trump did not allow. The loss of high-paying jobs related to the shutdown of the Keystone pipeline and other fossil fuel-related projects put workers and related businesses in unsustainable positions, something unforeseen by many prior to the election.

Another side effect of the pandemic's ability to change the voting system was empowering those who canceled the *Remain in Mexico* policy put in place by then U.S. President Trump, which effectively opened the US southern border to a flood of millions of undocumented and often COVID-19-positive immigrants from countries within and outside the Americas. This open border policy allowed over a million illegal immigrants entry into the US by the middle of 2021. Some argued the cancelation was an attempt by the newly elected government to increase the number of voters who would support the political party that allowed them access and help them remain in power. While this attempt to further secure their tenure as the political party in power served its intended purpose, it also created a potentially dangerous situation for businesses due to increased criminal activity by Mexican and South American drug cartels, illegal immigrants who had no legal source of income, and violent criminal organizations such as MS13.

7. Mortality Rates and the Side Effects of Lockdowns

While government-mandated lockdowns were the norm in the US and other European countries, countries like Nigeria discovered that lockdown strategies could worsen the spread of the virus under certain situations due to poor management and a lack of facilities (Baba et al. 2021). Coccia's (2021a, 2021b) study addressed the relationship between the length of lockdowns, the numbers of infected people and fatalities attributed to COVID-19, and the negative economic impact of such extended measures. The findings revealed there were no reductions in the spread or mortality of the virus associated with extended lockdowns as opposed to shorter lockdowns and conversely showed significant negative disruptions to economic growth and stability. Statisticians continue to argue over whether masks and isolation are effective in limiting the spread of the virus yet admit there has not been enough experience to fully understand why some areas fare better than others with fewer restrictions (Curley 2021).

The confusion regarding mortality rates provides a way for politicians, media sources, medical experts, and internet pundits to exploit ignorance in support of their various agendas. Crude mortality rates, case fatality rates (CFR), and infection fatality rates (IFR) are often treated as synonymous, yet they are calculated very differently and imply vastly different perspectives on the true risk of dying from COVID-19. The crude mortality rate is the number of confirmed deaths by a specific cause divided by the total population even those who were never infected. Using such a number is misleading because it does not provide potential victims with their chances for survival. Case fatality rates are likewise flawed in that it divides the number of confirmed deaths from a specific cause by the number who were diagnosed as being infected while far greater numbers may have contracted the illness went undiagnosed due to being either asymptomatic or having only minor symptoms that did not warrant a visit to a doctor or hospital. Infection fatality rates are a true measure of the lethality of an illness; however, due to the potential for large portions of a population being undiagnosed, the IFR can only be calculated if the entire population is tested for the illness; a study not yet conducted (Ritchie et al. 2021). As a result of this situation, those who wish to justify extreme measures cite the CFR, and those who oppose such measures cite the crude mortality rate to support their opposing position.

Expert opinion on how the pandemic would unfold and its long-term effects were often incorrect or based on too little information and consideration for the public's desire to return to previous norms. Hochmann (2020) argued that the pandemic would change everything from how we greet one another to how the public would fixate on washing away deadly germs. The 73% increase in sales of sanitizers in March 2020 accompanied a U.S. government order for hundreds of millions of N95 masks despite Dr. Fauci's earlier statements that masks were a placebo rather than an effective prevention of virus spread. The shift from handshake greetings to elbow bumping was predicted to be the new normal, and while such behavior is not uncommon in 2021, there are many who still extend a hand rather than an elbow. However, most stores how have sanitizing stations installed at their entrance to accommodate those who still fear a virus that studies have shown are unlikely to be transmitted on surfaces. Perceptions confused by changing information, misinformation, and erroneous predictions have created divisions in the population that affect how business is conducted and offices are managed. Perception, or the management of perception, is critical. A 2020 study in Romania was performed with a 719-sample size of adults aged 18–75 years. A review of the collected data indicated the younger members of the study considered the risk of COVID-19 infection was moderate. Although these younger members questioned the restrictions, they subsequently followed their government's guidance on sanitation and social distancing, considering such guidance as supporting the needs of the Romanian community (Matei et al. 2021). This is in contrast with the perceptual politicization of measures within the US, where the federal mandates often conflict with the perceptions of individual state governments. These differences suggest an added layer of consideration and frustration of businesses that conduct operations across national and state borders.

All these factors show that a global event, whether it be a pandemic, volcanic eruptions, major earthquake, or mass migration, can have unpredictable effects on businesses and governments. The event itself will have immediate and long-term consequences, yet the disruption created by the event will allow marginalized and radical elements to rise to power or influence that can have an even greater effect on the business environment, global supply chains, and worker expectations. Workers look to their leaders, whether those leaders be in government or the workplace, to keep them safe and secure. Unexpected global events make support and guidance of those workers more challenging, especially when there is not a plan in place prior to the event. Businesses, and governments, need to better plan for disruptive or catastrophic events if they are to continue with any sort of continuity. Without such planning, the resulting chaos could so change the environment as to make the new normal something previously inconceivable.

8. How to Prepare for the Next Global Disruption?

Preparation for an unexpected global disruption may seem an impossible task. Details of the unexpected are not always foreseeable, yet each will affect certain business processes. Although specific disruptions may or may not be predictable from a *when* perspective, most are predictable by a *what* perspective and perhaps even result in generic responses that would cover a wide range of business practice and supply chain disruptions. Wang et al. (2021) responded to a Verschuur et al. (2021) critical analysis of their predictions regarding estimated disruptions to global supply chains. The response to the critique posited that it was not possible to compare the stylized lockdown scenarios with data reflecting actual changes in the economy due to unpredictable policy changes, adding that Verschuur et al.'s data had limitations on how well it reflected changes to global supply chains and how it only reflected a specific part of international trade. Wang et al. further explained that they did not aim to predict the true cost of COVID-19, only possible consequences under different types of lockdown scenarios, none of which occurred exactly as modeled. The article by Wang et al., the critical analysis by Verschuur et al., and the response to that analysis indicate the limitations involved by even the most sophisticated analysts when it comes to unexpected global disruptions.

9. Job Loss and An Accelerated Shift to Virtual Offices

Reactions to the COVID-19 pandemic were varied with millions losing their job and others learning to work from home (BBC 2020). Some businesses were already working in a virtual environment, which meant having to stay at home was not a real issue as far as work production or service provision was concerned. Other businesses were fully reliant on physical attendance in the workplace. These businesses had to scramble in efforts to find ways to continue to work in a new environment. The technology existed yet had not been implemented or configured for the work required by the business's employees. In some cases, the workers were too unfamiliar with the technologies that would allow virtual work; in other cases, the businesses felt they had to reduce the workforce or production levels, which in turn affected the supply chain to which they were a functional part. Other businesses had already established a hybrid workforce of on-site and remote workers and were, therefore, able to more readily adapt to the new conditions. Had not such a large portion of businesses been able to conduct their business in a virtual/work-from-home environment, world economies would have collapsed during the extended lockdowns (Wong 2020).

One perhaps unexpected result of allowing employees to work from home was the realization that more than half found working at home preferable to working in the office with more flexible hours, a better balance of work and family responsibilities with some reporting they had higher productivity in a virtual environment. An analysis of the workforce in eight countries suggested 20%–25% of the workforce in advanced economies could work from home between three and five days per week, and a survey of 278 executives by McKinsey in August 2020 predicted a 30% reduction in office space (Lund et al. 2021). Deguchi (2020) suggested there would not be a return to the old business model in Japan, arguing that the pandemic accelerated the move toward a paperless society and an end to the 2-hour commute for many of Tokyo's 40 million people living in the greater Tokyo metropolitan area. A report from the US Bureau of Labor Statistics (Dey et al. 2020) estimated 31% of the workers employed in early March of 2020 had switched to teleworking from home by the first week of April. Lister, president of Global Workplace Analytics, forecasted 25%–30% of the workforce will still be working from home by the end of 2021 (2020).

Stewart Butterfield, CEO and founder of Slack, indicated the experience of having workers perform their duties from home has provided an opportunity to retain the best parts of office culture while eliminating bad habits and processes, such as ineffective meetings and an unnecessary bureaucracy. Butterfield also posited that people are now making new choices about where they want to live and how they want to work. They have new expectations about flexibility and working choices with 72% of 4,700 workers surveyed indicating they never wanted to go back to the old model of working in an office, preferring to work in a hybrid model going forward (Arvedlund 2020; BBC 2020; Parker et al. 2020). Another third indicated they would prefer to work from home at least some of the time with a small share who wanted to go back to the office full time (Averlund 2020). There was a 23%–31%split between women and men who would prefer to work from home, whether or not children were involved. This split in turn raised the question as to whether working from home would improve gender equality (BBC 2020). This was not the case for all workers, however, as approximately 62% of American jobs cannot be done from home with Melinda Gates citing a study that found women were 1.8 times more likely to lose their job than men (BBC 2020), showing a gender and class divide between those who can and those who cannot work from home. Those who can work from home generally have college degrees with about two-thirds who hold a bachelor's degree or higher. Of the remainder who can work from home, approximately 23%, do not hold a college degree. Meanwhile, according to the Pew Research Center, the majority of middle and lower-income workers cannot work from home (Averlund 2020). Microsoft (2021) held a US hybrid work summit on September 29, 2021, in which the speakers included the president of Microsoft US, several Microsoft corporate vice presidents, Forrester Research, and Rex Miller, a futurologist and author. The focus of the summit was to present key trends in the shift to a hybrid workforce, how to reimagine businesses with a new operating model that supports hybrid work, and the potential evolution of hybrid work.

These figures and the Microsoft summit represent and address a significant liability for businesses that rely heavily on those who cannot work from home should conditions arise that prevent an *on-site* workforce. Elisabeth Reynolds, executive director of MIT's task force on the work of the future, cited the greatest challenge to be faced is what to do with the 60% of workers who cannot work from home (BBC 2020). Government, public administration, and military workforces are almost equally divided between those who can and cannot work from home with about 46% indicating they could work from home.

Meanwhile, around three-quarters of those in the retail, trade, or transportation industry (84%); manufacturing, mining, construction, agriculture, forestry, fishing/hunting (78%); and hospitality, service, arts, entertainment, and recreation (77%); and about 66% of those in the health care and social assistance sector cannot work from home. Those in public-facing positions, such as restaurant workers, healthcare, police and fire, and waste management, by the very nature of their job, are unable to work from home. Those who cannot work from home and are in critical positions are more concerned with the potential of infecting other family members, which in turn adds additional stress above what results from other pandemic concerns (Averlund 2020). Brownell (2020) indicated a shift in office design to accommodate social distancing or de-densification is becoming a new consideration as businesses plan on returning those who cannot work remotely to an office environment. Some of these changes include the erection of space-dividing partitions, rotating schedules (PwC 2021), and greater separation of workstations. These considerations are making some businesses consider finding ways to reduce their physical footprint by finding new ways for employees to accomplish their work remotely. Some experts believe businesses should consider employing a community manager to function as the connective tissue between on-site and remote employees and as a business ambassador for the company's brand and culture while monitoring trends and requests to further increase the businesses' flexibility and productivity as a hybrid workplace (Schneider 2020). Future office models may also look to digital solutions focused on *touch-free* interfaces, such as voice recognition in elevators, motion sensors, virtual assistants, and mobile applications to allow employee interaction without the risk of cross-contamination (STO Building Group 2020).

Businesses must also contend with contradictory situations, such as whether it is better to isolate individuals or consider allowing them to work together. A study conducted by Sheldon Cohen determined that isolated employees are three times more likely to catch a virus than those who many close contacts with others. This, however, is in contradiction to CDC guidelines that advocate social distancing, banning assemblies, avoiding face-to-face situations, and chance encounters (Brownell 2020). The same holds true for adolescents whose suicide rate increased when in-class education shifted to remote learning. Businesses, including colleges and universities, must constantly weigh the latest revisions to laws, guidelines, and corporate policies to ensure they provide a safe working environment, within the law and in the best interests of their students and workforce while avoiding litigation based on a perceived threat to worker health or well-being (Kapasia et al. 2020).

Regardless of whether a business could accommodate a virtual workforce, the workers still expect guidance from their employers. Fear of reductions in force, mortgage defaults resulting from reduced hours or unemployment, loss of medical coverage, cost of food and services were all realities that had to be faced by workers who continued to look to their employers for answers. Larger social issues created by governmental restrictions or policies were not really the responsibility of employers, yet employees often asked their employer for guidance. Businesses responded based on their knowledge of changes to local, state, and federal laws, mandates by the CDC and other nongovernmental agencies, unions, and media forces. Some businesses felt obligated to succumb to radical media pressure and change corporate logos, policies, venues, and hiring practices. Other businesses chose to maintain the status quo and risk social media ridicule, shaming or ostracizing for not complying with such pressures. The canceling of positions, individuals, and organizations fueled the fear of standing a business's ground, resulting in capitulation by those who relied heavily on perception and social media exposure. Businesses must carefully consider how to address changing guidance and issues to retain their identity without risking the loss of business. Businesses may not want to risk lower worker retention or business closure because they decide not to conform to new norms or expectations. The solution may be found in how the new ruling party deals with difficult questions and situations that change the narrative.

10. How to Comply Without Really Trying?

A business does not need to necessarily comply if they simply do not focus on their differences. Remaining neutral in such situations can be achieved by providing an answer that does not answer the question. For example, if a business is asked what is being done to make itself more equitable, they can respond by saying, "We have always embraced equity in the workforce and are a leader in our industry in this regard." If they are asked what policies they have in place to ensure equity, they can simply say, "Our policies are inherently focused on equity at all levels." Specifics are not as important as the appearance of answering the question, without hesitation, and using sound bites that appear to address the question in a positive light. If another difficult question is asked in response to the previous answer, simply provide the previous answer, and move on. Anyone who thinks such a response will not work should pay more attention to responses by government officials who routinely use this tactic during press conferences.

11. How to Prepare for the Unexpected?

What can a business do to prepare for the unexpected? There are only a few variables to consider regardless of the type of unexpected global event. First and foremost is to identify how the business currently does business and how certain disruptions might be handled. For example, for a business currently without virtual workers, how might they modify their business model to allow at least a portion of the workforce to be virtual? Indranil Roy, executive director for Deloitte Consulting, argued that businesses can probably accomplish most tasks remotely without a significant drop in productivity or quality. However, in the long term, face-to-face interaction is required to support collaboration, relationship building, and solve complex problems while continuous remote work extends the workday and reduces mental well-being. Roy promoted the idea of a virtual-first model where the workplace is distributed across the home, office, and satellite offices to allow a flexible choice of how the workforce interacts (BBC 2020). For the balance of the workforce, what training would have to be provided to ensure their continued work in a virtual environment? In other words, move those who can be moved to a virtual environment when it is not required and train those who are unfamiliar or unprepared to move to a virtual environment. Training is a key factor as a study of Italian workers noted that remote workers must be competent in remote tools or risk decreases in productivity. Additionally, those who cannot work with autonomy are not familiar with communication tools or are unable to keep productive relationships with remote peers due to unfamiliarity with these tools will be less productive (Bolisani et al. 2020). This training must therefore include educating the workforce on how to use video communications to ensure continuity and familiarity with business partners and peers. Eric Yuan, founder and CEO of Zoom, one of a few popular video communication solutions, suggested businesses are growing and improving with the help of video communication. This new exposure to video communication has helped numerous industries stay connected to a point where such communication is often considered commonplace (BBC 2020).

Another consideration is the monitoring and control of remote workers. Businesses relatively inexperienced with managing remote workers need to learn how to effectively motivate, reward, and interact with their workers in new ways using new tools. However, experts believe there are risks associated with the misuse of these tools and cite data indicating that they are being misused. Surveillance tools, enforcing protocols, ensuring productivity while safeguarding against legal liability, all provide businesses information, yet that information often provides an incomplete picture of worker productivity and compliance. There are risks of privacy infringement and backlashes to business executives from employee concerns generated by increased monitoring, demands for constant communication, and an oversimplification of productivity assessment (Nguyen 2020). There is an inherent risk of misunderstanding and misuse of metrics associated with productivity. Nguyen (2020) cited a situation noted by journalist Adam Satariano who subjected himself and his boss to a work surveillance program called Hubstaff for three weeks. The metrics from this program suggested there was a 50% decrease in his productivity by basing his performance on typing and mouse movement while not considering phone calls and other noncomputer work. Managers using such surveillance software must understand Albert Einstein's blackboard warning that "not everything that counts can be counted, and not everything that can be counted counts."

Video communication works well at the managerial and remote worker levels, but what if the business's product requires physical presence? While video communication might serve to keep distant workers connected on a social or team level, it will not allow physical action at a distance. So how might businesses adapt? One possible solution might be to change working hours to provide access to the same number of workers but on different shifts to minimize the number of workers present at any point in time. Another option might be to automate certain processes that are monitored or controlled remotely. What would such a modification cost? How few products can a business produce and remain profitable? How can they assist other members of their supply chain to ensure no or limited disruption during such events?

12. What about Supply Chains?

Few businesses operate completely independent of a supply chain even if a part of that supply chain is the power to their facilities. Businesses, large or small, must remain aware of supply chain volatility, uncertainty, complexity, and ambiguity (VUCA) and turbulent, uncertain, novel, and ambiguous (TUNA) changes regardless of the underlying environmental reasons (Gordon 2018). Most large businesses have backup power, yet that backup is usually not sufficient to keep up full production. The question then becomes, what happens if you lose power? Additionally, what happens if you lose internet connectivity? What happens if the entire internet goes down? How vulnerable is your system to ransomware? How diversified and accessible is your data? How would you conduct business if the roads were closed? How automated is your business? How vulnerable are your supply chain members? What happens if there is an interruption in cell phone service? What options do you have for supply support? For example, some businesses have a major supplier and others that are less cost-effective but provide alternative support should a major supplier have an interruption in service. These businesses believe the extra cost is worth the flexibility and risk reduction.

The bottom line is that businesses need to address supply chain and operational vulnerabilities by having a reaction plan that covers virtually all scenarios. Various frameworks exist to better prepare organizations to more rapidly react to supply chain disturbances. A business or organization must first manage the fundamental business processes and inventory management that support workflow and information transparency. They must then ensure they understand how they are networked and connected via their factories, delivery, distribution, and external communication. Communication, physical supply, workforce capability in a physical or virtual environment, data collection, access, and transfer, power requirements, and physical access are all considerations. For example, Texas uses fossil fuel, solar, and wind-powered electrical generation systems. However, a severe snowstorm in 2021 froze the wind turbines and blocked out the sun. The cold weather situation required increased electricity for heating since the state had moved away from fossil fuels for heating. The loss of electrical generation capacity, coupled with increased demand for power resulted in homes going without heat during rolling blackouts. While Texas had seemingly increased its diversity of power generation, it relied on the combined capability of all generation sources without considering environmental situations that could reduce one or more of those sources. This same flaw in business planning can be seen in almost all industries. It is, therefore, imperative that an organization or business understands the macro level of their supply chain and how social and natural environmental changes inherently create risks which require prior planning to ensure resilience in their supply chains. The inability to obtain a single computer chip can impact production in the automobile industry, reminding supply chain managers that disruption of even such an apparent minor part in a complex system can halt, delay, or otherwise impact production.

13. What Now?

Unexpected events may be short-lived or linger and morph into ongoing situations that require organizations and businesses to balance uncertainty on the one hand and sustainability on the other.

Earthquakes and other natural disasters are often disruptive yet short-lived. Viral outbreaks were previously perceived as short-lived, yet the recent COVID-19 pandemic appears to have a longer lifespan as governments continue to shift positions when variations of the virus emerge. Whether the reactions by governments are justified or overblown, the effects to supply chains and business processes are real. These political and social vacillations create havoc to businesses as they open, close, reopen, and try to maintain a workforce who might rather stay home and receive compensation than return to work for less money or the risk of infection. Government compensations to businesses are notoriously biased, whether in favor of certain majorities or minorities or by business type. Those businesses flagged as critical infrastructure are equally capriciously assigned. In the case of opening or closing schools, the science indicated young children were not carriers or in danger of infection, yet teachers' unions refused to go back to work until the buildings were modified and all children were vaccinated. Even when forced to go back to school, children were forced to wear masks even though the science indicated the wearing of masks posed a greater threat to their health than the virus.

Fear is a little mind killer and ignorance fans the flame of actions that may be counterproductive or even harmful. What do governments or businesses do when medical experts cannot agree or reverse their stance on how the public should react? Who makes the call that weighs the benefits associated with forced closures, masked students, unemployed workers, and the collapse of an economy against the potential threat of death or infection? From a medical position, it's all about protecting a population from infection regardless of the socioeconomic impact on the population. Such a one-sided view ignores the reality that preventing infection at the cost of losing your home, your ability to buy food, or the social trauma isolation brings. The ability of governments to manipulate such situations to promote their own agenda is real and unavoidable. The only action businesses can take is to remain nimble and adaptable to ever-changing restrictions.

14. The Chain Effect and the New Normal

Regardless of how well a business plans for unexpected events, others in their supply chain could be affected in unexpected ways. In a global economy with supply chains stretching around the world, a course of action in one country could adversely affect a business in another that relies on an unbroken supply chain. In other words, a business can only control so much, especially when the supply chain involves businesses in other countries. No plan is perfect yet planning for unexpected disruptions is possible. The choice to stockpile a greater inventory of material sourced outside the control of a business located in another country comes at a cost that must be subjected to risk analysis. Too large a stockpile could result in inventory that becomes obsolete or expired before its use. Using multiple suppliers located in different parts of the world might increase resiliency yet result in increased costs by keeping supply lines open from a higher-cost supplier. The chain effect of a business disrupted by a single part unreceived in its supply chain ripples down to those expecting a part they deliver, which further disrupts the chain for those relying on their parts or services. Adding to the situation is the reality that some parts come from a single country or business provider. If that business relies on raw material from a country impacted by a natural disaster or government change, the entire supply chain is affected.

The business world is networked across dozens, sometimes hundreds, of supply lines, each one vulnerable to a host of issues, expected and unexpected. The *new normal* is never cast in stone and it is perhaps better to forget the thought of normalcy and understand that there is only the *now* and the projected *future* when it comes to operational models. There are simply too many variables to consider anything as static stability; the only reliable model is one that is ready for constant change. The new normal, therefore, does not exist outside of *normal* meaning model instability and the need for resilience and adaptability to an ever-changing environment. The recent pandemic has made this abundantly clear, and organizations and businesses can either accept this reality or fight against situations beyond their control. Galloway (2020) warned that businesses should not trust the free market to sort the way ultra-large technical businesses behave in a post-pandemic world because they are an unnatural, unregulated system with no moral compass. It will ultimately be up to governments and the general population to ensure the future is symbiotic and not parasitic to the general population.

15. Chief Concerns of Business Managers

Gray (2020) compiled a list of concerns expressed by managers related to remote working. The list addressed concerns over productivity, technology, employee perspectives, security, and strategy. These concerns were over the positive and negative effects of remote working. For example, regarding productivity, while productivity increased, so did the number of overtime hours worked including work on the weekends. On technology, over half of the employees indicated their employer needed to invest in better technology with nearly 40% indicating they had to partially or fully fund their required upgrades. Even among IT teams, 37% indicated they did not have the right tools, and 43% experienced issues with multifactor authentication while dealing with an insecure, undersized virtual private network. In relation to employee perspectives, 98% of those surveyed indicated a desire to work from home for the rest of their careers with 93% indicating they would like to work remotely at least some of the time. The 62% of those surveyed indicated they would actually take a cut in pay to work from home; the 78% would be willing to take a 5% cut in pay with 20% willing to take a 10% cut in pay.

The study's findings on security-related concerns, an issue for any business with remote workers, revealed over 10% of the employees had their video calls hacked, 46% noted an increase in phishing attacks, and 46% of global businesses have encountered at least one cybersecurity scare since the start of the pandemic. These realities translate into a need to shift and reshape business strategies, especially in the technical priorities. Businesses now expect that nearly 40% of their employees will use a remote working model in a post-pandemic world. Seventy-five percent of executives agreed that digital transformation has become a more urgent priority with 78% believing digital employees are both essential and a high priority as opposed to only 49% prior to the pandemic.

How much a business spends on moving part or all its workforce to a virtual environment depends on the nature of the business and the risks they are willing to take in a future that at times defies prediction. Ultimately, businesses will need to increase their flexibility, adaptability, and forecasting ability, all while finding ways to manage a hybrid workforce that may be dispersed around the world. Virtual workforces cannot operate if there is a disruption to the internet, so what provision has a business made to either return to an on-site model or find another way to manage remote operations? On-site production can be disrupted by local environmental events, such as earthquakes, tornadoes, hurricanes, or political unrest; what provisions have been made to ensure disrupted work or supply chain support can be shifted or otherwise transferred to another location?

Each business will need to engage in *what-if* scenario planning, whether based on historical events or wild imaginings. Businesses that fail to plan for the unexpected will ultimately have to adjust without a plan and risk total business collapse. The food industry witnessed the closure of many restaurants while others were able to shift to a delivery service to stay in business. However, others who should have been able to shift to a delivery model were unable to do so because their supply chain was disrupted, and it took too long to find other options. A business can only survive if it can adapt, and adaptation is more difficult if prior planning is not part of the business model. As Benjamin Franklin may have stated, "By failing to prepare you are preparing to fail." Whether the quote can be accurately attributed to him or not, the message is clear: Make advance plans or risk being unable to adapt quickly enough to survive. There are no guarantees other than the certainty that business environments and the rules under which they operate will continue to change, often in unexpected ways and within shorter periods of time. In the words of German military strategist Helmuth von Moltke who in 1871 wrote, "No plan of operations extends with any certainty beyond the first encounter with the main enemy forces." Put into a business perspective, *no contingency plan will remain unchanged after first application during a crisis.* The point is this, plans are necessary, yet so is a business's ability to adapt those plans to changing circumstances as they are put into action. Without a plan, a starting point, there is only chaos and confusion where decisions are made at a time where clear thinking is abandoned to emotional intuition.

References

"A timeline of COVID-19 developments in 2020." *American Journal of Managed Care.* https://www.ajmc.com/view/a-timeline-of-covid19-developments-in-2020

Atalan, A. 2020. "Is the lockdown important to prevent the COVID-19 pandemic? Effects on psychology, environment and economy-perspective." *Annals of Medicine and Surgery,* 56 (August): 38–42. https://doi.org/10.1016/j.amsu.2020.06.010

Arvedlund, E. 2020. "Working from home is a hit: Most WFH Americans want to keep teleworking after COVID-19." *Chicago Tribune* (December 14). https://www.chicagotribune.com/business/ct-biz-working-from-home-pandemic-survey-20201214-zvzsborfrng lfnv6trcexzvmrq-story.html

Baba, I. A., Yusuf, A., Nisar, K. S., Abdel-Aty, A. H., and Nofal, T. A. 2021. "Mathematical model to assess the imposition of lockdown during COVID-19 pandemic." *Results in Physics,* 20 (January). https://doi.org/10.1016/j.rinp.2020.103716

BBC. 2020. "Coronavirus: How the world of work may change forever." *BBC Worklife.* https://www.bbc.com/worklife/article/20201023-coronavirus-how-will-the-pandemic-change-the-way-we-work

Bolisani, E., Scarso, E., Ipsen, C., Kirchner, K., and Hansen, J. P. 2020. "Working from home during COVID-19 pandemic: Lessons learned and issues." *Management and Marketing,* 15 (1): 458–476. https://doi.org/10.2478/mmcks-2020-0027

Brownell, B. 2020. "Rethinking office design trends in a post-COVID world." *Architect* (May 18). https://www.architectmagazine. com/practice/rethinking-office-design-trends-in-a-post-covid-world o

Centers for Disease Control and Prevention (CDC). (2021, December 1). SARS-Vov-2 variant classifications and definitions. https://www. cdc.gov/coronavirus/2019-ncov/variants/variant-classifications.html

Coccia, M. 2021a. "Effects of a longer duration of lockdown on COVID-19 related infected individuals and deaths, and on economic growth of countries." *Science of the Total Environment, 775* (February 24). https://doi.org/10.1016/j.scitotenv.2021.145801

Coccia, M. 2021b. "The relation between length of lockdown, numbers of infected people and deaths of COVID-19, and economic growth of countries: Lessons learned to cope with future pandemics similar to COVID-19 and to constrain the deterioration of economic system." *Science of the Total Environment, 775* (June 21). https://doi.org/10.1016/j.scitotenv.2021.145801

Curley, C. 2021. "Why do California and Florida have similar COVID-19 case rates? The answer is complicated." *Healthline* (February 21). https://www.healthline.com/health-news/why-do-california-and-florida-have-similar-covid-19-case-rates-the-answer-is-complicated

Deguchi, H. 2020. "The new normal that will arise after COVID-19." *The Japan Times* (November 22). https://www.japantimes.co.jp/opinion/2020/11/22/commentary/japan-commentary/new-normal-coronavirus/

Dey, M., Frazis, H., Loewenstein, M. A., and Sun, H. 2020. "Ability to work from home: evidence from two surveys and implications for the labor market in the COVID-19 pandemic." *U.S. Bureau of Labor Statistics* (June). https://www.bls.gov/opub/mlr/2020/article/ability-to-work-from-home.htm

Galloway, S., and Kennelly, D. 2020. "Post-Covid and the new normal." *City Journal* (November 30). https://www.city-journal.org/post-covid-and-new-normal

Gordon, A. V. 2018. "You say VUCA, I say TUNA: How Oxford helps leaders face the complex and uncertain future." *Forbes* (January 19). https://www.forbes.com/sites/adamgordon/2016/04/06/oxford/?sh=61c555cd4314

Gray, R. 2020. "74 statistics on remote working during COVID-19 lockdown." *Wandera* (July 21). https://www.wandera.com/statistics-on-remote-working-during-covid-19-lockdown/

Hochman, D. 2020. "The new normal: What comes after COVID-19?" *AARP* (June 8). https://www.aarp.org/health/conditions-treatments/info-2020/daily-life-after-pandemic-predictions.html

Jiang, P., Klemeš, J. J., Fan, Y. V., Fu, X., and Bee, Y. M. 2021. "More Is Not Enough: A Deeper Understanding of the COVID-19 Impacts on Healthcare, Energy and Environment Is Crucial." *International Journal of Environmental Research and Public Health, 18*(2), 684. https://doi.org/10.3390/ijerph18020684

Johnson, D. J., Tress, T., Burkel, N., Taylor, C., and Cesario, J. 2019. "Officer characteristics and racial disparities in fatal officer-involved shootings." *Proceedings of the National Academy of Sciences of the United States of America,* 116 (32) (August 6). https://doi.org/10.1073/pnas.1903856116

Kapasia, N., Paul, P., Roy, A., Saha, J., Zaveri, A., Mallick, R., Barman, B., Das, P., and Chouhan, P. 2020. "Impact of lockdown on learning status of undergraduate and postgraduate students during COVID-19 pandemic in West Bengal, India." *Children and Youth Services Review,* 116 (September). https://doi.org/10.1016/j.childyouth.2020.105194

Katella, K. 2021. "5 things to know about the Delta variant: The predominant COVID-19 strain has put the focus back on prevention." *Yale Medicine* (November 19). https://www.yalemedicine.org/news/5-things-to-know-delta-variant-covid

King, N. (Host), Allen, G., and Westervelt, E. 2021. "Pandemic approaches: The differences between Florida, California." *NPR*

(February 18) https://www.npr.org/2021/02/18/968921902/ pandemic-approaches-the-differences-between-florida-california

Lister, K. 2020. "Work-at-home after COVID-19—Our forecast." *Global Workplace Analytics*. Retrieved November 1, 2021. https://global workplaceanalytics.com/work-at-home-after-covid-19-our-forecast

Live Science Staff. (2021, December 10). Coronavirus variants: Facts about omicron, delta and other COVID-19 mutants. https://www.livescience.com/coronavirus-variants.html

Lund, S., Madgavkar, A., Manyika, J., Smit, S., Ellingrud, K., Meaney, M., and Robinson, O. 2021. *The Future of Work after COVID-19* (February 18). McKinsey & Company. https://www.mckinsey.com/featured-insights/future-of-work/the-future-of-work-after-covid-19

Matei, E., Ilovan, O., Sandu, C., Dumitrache, L., Istrate, M., Jucu, I., and Gavrilidis, A. 2021. "Early COVID-19 pandemic impacts on society and environment in Romania. Perception among population with higher education." *Environmental Engineering and Management Journal*, 20 (2): 319–330. http://eemj.eu/index.php/EEMJ/article/view/4283

Mac Donald, H. 2020. "The myth of systemic police racism." *Wall Street Journal* (September 2). https://www.wsj.com/articles/the-myth-of-systemic-police-racism-11591119883

Masoud, N., and Bohra, O. P. 2020. "Challenges and opportunities of distance learning during COVID-19 in UAE." *Academy of Accounting and Financial Studies Journal*, 24 (1): 1–12. https://search.proquest.com/openview/f558c90e3d1325852348a2d7157 7cf98/1?pq-origsite=gscholarandcbl=29414

Mucci, F., Mucci, N., and Diolaiuti, F. 2020. "Lockdown and isolation: Psychological aspects of COVID-19 pandemic in the general population." *Clinical Neuropsychiatry,* 17 (2): 63–64. https://delphicentre.com.au/uploads/01.%20App%20-%20 Attachment%202020/5.%202020-02-02-Muccietal.pdf

Microsoft. 2021. "Microsoft US Hybrid Work Summit." Retrieved September 8, 2021. https://mktoevents.com/ Microsoft+Event/288772/157-GQE-382

Njolomole, M. 2020. "States that stayed open fared much better than states that shut down." *Center of the American Experiment* (August 27). https://www.americanexperiment.org/2020/08/states-that-stayed-open-fared-much-better-than-states-that-shut-down/

Nguyen, A. 2020. "On the clock and at home: Post-COVID-19 employee monitoring in the workplace." *SHRM Executive Network.* https:// www.shrm.org/executive/resources/people-strategy-journal/ summer2020/Pages/feature-nguyen.aspx

Parker, K., Horowitz, J. M., and Minkin, R. 2020. "How the Coronavirus outbreak has—and hasn't—changed the way Americans work." *Pew Research Center* (December 9). https://www.pewresearch. org/social-trends/2020/12/09/how-the-coronavirus-outbreak-has-and-hasnt-changed-the-way-americans-work/

PwC. 2021. *It's Time to Reimagine Where and How Work Will Get Done* (January 12). https://www.pwc.com/us/en/library/covid-19/us-remote-work-survey.html

Ritchie, H., Ortiz-Ospina, E., Beltekian, D., Mathieu, E., Hasell, J., Macdonald, B., Giattino, C., Appel, C., and Roser, M. 2021. "Statistics and research: Mortality risk of COVID-19." *Our World in Data* (March 9). Retrieved March 9, 2021. https:// ourworldindata.org/mortality-risk-covid

Schneider, A. 2020,. "4 design trends of a post-COVID workplace." *Interior Design* (July 22). https://www.interiordesign.net/articles/18254-4-design-trends-of-a-post-covid-workplace/

STO Building Group. 2020. *The Post COVID Workplace: What's Next for Office Design?* (September 22). https://structuretone.com/the-post-covid-workplace-whats-next-for-office-design/

The Editorial Board. 2020. "News from the non-lockdown states: Per-capita Covid fatalities were 75% lower in open states." *The Wall Street Journal* (June 23). https://www.wsj.com/articles/news-from-the-non-lockdown-states-11592954700

The Poynter Institute. 2021 "Due to differing lockdown orders, New York has more COVID-19 cases, deaths, hospitalizations and job losses than Florida, and New York also lags on vaccinations." *PolitiFact* (February 26). https://www.politifact.com/factchecks/2021/feb/26/instagram-posts/chart-comparing-new-york-and-florida-covid-19-flaw/

Verschuur, J., Koks, E. E., and Hall, J. W. 2021. "Observed impacts of the COVID-19 pandemic on global trade." *Nature Human Behavior 5* (February 25): 305–307. https://doi.org/10.1038/s41562-021-01060-5

Wang, D., Hubacek, K., Liang, X., Coffman, D., Hallegatte, S., and Guan, D. 2021. "Reply to: Observed impacts of the COIVD-19 pandemic on global trade." *Nature Human Behavior* (February 25). https://doi.org/10.1038/s41562-021-01061-4

Wong, M. 2020. "Standford research provides a snapshot of a new working-from-home economy." *Standford News* (June 29). https://news.stanford.edu/2020/06/29/snapshot-new-working-home-economy/

World Health Organization (WHO). 2021. *Update on Omicron* (November 28). https://www.who.int/news/item/28-11-2021-update-on-omicron

World Health Organization (WHO). (2022, January 10). Tracking SARS-CoV-2 variants. https://www.who.int/en/activities/tracking-SARS-CoV-2-variants/

Yang, E. 2020. "A closer look at the states that stayed open." *American Institute for Economic Research* (August 24)

CHAPTER 3

Impact of COVID-19 on Global Gig Economy

by A. C. Brahmbhatt

Abstract

The gig economy sector is the sector that comprises of part-time, temporary, and freelance jobs. It is also referred to as sharing economy sector or collaborative economy sector, where individuals can market their skill sets on different online platforms. COVID-19 with its widespread devastation in almost all spheres of life the world over has unsettled the global gig economy sector too. India's gig economic sector is significantly impacted by it. This chapter attempts to study the current scenario in the gig economy of the countries like USA, UK, China, Brazil, Japan, and India. The chapter provides a critical evaluation of the efficacy of change management strategies adopted by some countries like direct cash payments or *stimulus checks* to gig workers in response to the pandemic, modifications in their existing labor laws.

The COVID-19 has almost ravaged this sector, yet some companies, such as Uber, Airbnb, Zomato, HopSkipDrive, and others remained anti-fragile by providing efficient services at a cheaper rate. This chapter investigates the change management strategies adopted by such companies to safeguard against the damage caused by the pandemic.

A few pieces of evidence from economic research demonstrate some positive impacts of the COVID-19 pandemic, such as the increase in self-employment that is referred to as recession-pushed self-employment. As companies try to save costs, the demand for gig workers may spiral. Alternatively, if more people enter the gig economy to work flexibly, the competition even in gigs might increase. The countries also will have to devise strategies to deal with such competitive scenarios in the gig sector.

Keywords: Gig economy, anti-fragile, stimulus check, change management, pandemic, recession-pushed self-employment.

1. Introduction

A gig economy is a fragile economy with an agile workforce or a temporary workforce. It is a freelance economy. Originally coined in the 1920s by jazz musicians, the term is the short form of engagement. The gig works spread over a wide spectrum ranging from driving for Uber, delivering food, writing code to teaching as a part-time professor in some academic institute. Here the company is no longer an employer; it is a connector for contractors and clients. Employers who cannot afford full-time employees hire part-time workers. People who find making ends meet difficult in a turbulent time like the pandemic, need to do multiple jobs, preferably gig jobs. Those who have a fondness for changing careers, often those who enjoy flexibility also prefer to be a *gigger*. The gig workers do not have an advantage of health insurance, no medical leaves nor any maternity/paternity leaves and the gig work may turn out to be monotonous and stressful in the long run.

The pandemic has impacted different industries differently. For example, there is a steep rise in food groceries delivery services. But the ride services, restaurants, farmer markets, food truckers, gyms, spas, art industry are badly impacted. No official data or exhaustive information regarding the impact of COVID-19 on the global gig economy is available as yet. Several research teams in different universities/schools/agencies have started studying the phenomena in-depth, for example, Oxford University, Oxford Martin School, ADP Research Institute, and Statista. In the UK some research experts are engaged in the research work aiming at studying the impact of COVIB-19 on their gig economy.

Globally, the number of gig workers has increased by a marked extent. Gig economy accounts for a third of the world's working population and is expected to exceed the $500 billion mark in gross volume in the next five years (ADP Research Institute). The gig economy has the second-highest number of work opportunities offered. Approximately 68 million workers in the US work freelance and are projected to reach 90.1 million by 2028 (Statista Research Department 2021). Transportation–based services like ridesharing and carpooling platforms generate 58 percent of the gig economy's billion-dollar gross revenue. Fifty-nine percent of freelancers in the US are male, 40% female. Fifty-three percent of freelancers in the US are gazers or those aged 18–22 years old (Upwork 2020). The estimated total earnings of US-based, adult gig economy workers was $ 1.6 trillion in 2020. More than 50% of independent workers from different parts of the world are supplemental earners (daVinci Payments 2021).

In the study conducted by Upwork on the state of freelancing in 2020, the negative impact of the pandemic on existing freelancers was unveiled. According to it, 10% of US-based freelancers have paused freelancing at the onset of the pandemic. Twenty-eight percent of paused freelancers are either on leave or unemployed, and 51% still have other sources of work. Freelancing and remote work are perceived to be new trends reshaping future employment and business operations.

The regular workers now used to the work-from-home (WFH) model would find it difficult to go back to earlier 9–5 or 10–6 work schedule even after the pandemic.

OECD (2021) report has made some observations related to the impact of COVID-19 on the gig economy. According to it, it has impacted the activity of two large sectors of the gig economy—transportation (ride-sourcing) and short-term accommodation (real estate rental). Traditional businesses in sectors like restaurants that adopted technology-based distribution may continue using it even after the pandemic. The live-and-work-anywhere mindset that has grown up during the pandemic is likely to continue even after the pandemic.

The impact of COVID-19 on the gig economies of countries like the US, Canada, UK, Brazil, India, and the relief measures undertaken by them are discussed at length toward the later sections of the chapter.

1.1 Gig Economy

Gig economy is a free market system in which the companies enter into a short-term contract with independent workers. It is a freelance economy with an agile workforce or a temporary workforce. When people are fed up with conventional 9–5 office hours or 10–6 office hours, they prefer to be gigger. For a single employer, they balance various income streams and work independently job by job. Originally coined in 1920s by jazz musicians, the term is a short form of the word engagement.

A wide variety of jobs and positions fall into the category of a gig. It encompasses a wide spectrum, ranging from driving for Uber or delivering food to writing code or freelance articles. A gig worker can opt to work for a fixed number of hours, choosing a shift or work by project. Once the task or shift is complete, the gig worker move to the next gig—may be another task with the same company or something entirely different with another company. A gig worker may have a conventional day job (9–5 or 10–6) and then a second job at night.

In the gig economy, a company is not an employer; it is merely a connector, bringing contractors and clients together. Many companies that utilize gig workers, they do not employ them, for example, Uber, Instacart, TaskRabbit, Mechanical Turk.

- The factors responsible for a gig economy:

  The following are the probable factors responsible for a gig economy.

  - Employers who cannot afford to hire full-time employees to do all the necessary work will often hire part-time employees for the purpose.
  - From the employee's perspective, in order to afford their desired lifestyle, they need to take up multiple jobs.
  - There is a common tendency among people to change careers often during their lifetime. The gig-work is the reflection of such a tendency.
  - During COViD-19, those who have lost their regular jobs had to turn to part-time or contract jobs to earn their livelihood.

- The advantages and disadvantages of the gig economy.

The gig economy has certain advantages.

- Flexibility

  A gig worker is free to choose when or where she/he works, which clients she/he works for, what service/labor charges she/he demands from clients for the job done. The gig worker has the freedom to work on the days and timeslots of her/his choice.

  ii. Test-drive a new career

  The gig worker can test-drive different careers. If she/he loves baby grooming, she/he chooses to be a babysitter, loves pets, chooses to be a pet-sitter, even she/he can prefer to be a dog-walker.

  The gig economy has some disadvantages too.

- No health insurance, no medical leaves

  As a gig worker, she/he cannot get the benefit of health insurance, sick leaves, maternity/paternity leaves, travel allowance, etc., that are offered to the regular employees.

  ii. Becomes stressful

  Doing multiple jobs or the jobs at odd hours, in the long run, tells upon the health of the gig workers. Some jobs with no fixed time slots to do them become stressful and monotonous if continued for a longer period.

2.0 Impact of COVID-19 on Different Industries That Hire Gig Workers

COVID-19 has shattered the economies across the globe. Its first, second, and third wave in some countries have led to the crazy lockdown globally that has adversely impacted the big and small economies. Work from home (WFH) has become a new normal with an exponential rise in demand for gig workers as well. It has impacted different industries hiring gig workers differently. Some have seen a steep rise whereas some have witnessed a decline. For example, food-groceries delivery services have shown a steep rise as Work from Home (WFH) becoming new normal, people mostly do not move out of their homes. They order food and groceries online. Ride services, vis-à-vis this, experience a slowdown in their business. During the pandemic, people are frightened of the fact that it is very likely that the rider might be the carrier of the deadly virus. The demand for cabs and riders is very low due to the panic created by the coronavirus. That has adversely impacted the profits and ability of gig drivers to pay their bills.

It means there should be a substantial decline in the revenue for Uber and Lyft. But the reality is different. As they have adopted contractor business model, they are not much accountable to their employees and drivers, leaving drivers to their fate. The pandemic has generated such paradoxical scenarios too.

The governments and health professionals strictly enforced the COVID-appropriate behavior, such as social distancing, banning the large gathering, or canceling them. Even the people were instructed to stay safe at home and stock up on groceries. It had directly impacted restaurants, caterer's food truckers, farmer markets, gyms, spas, hairdressing salons, the entire art industry (theater, dance, paintings, books, etc.).

The event management industry is also no exception in suffering tremendous loss due to the pandemic. Hundreds of concerts, film premiers, music festivals, award-giving ceremonies, sports events, etc., were to be outright canceled, leaving producers, technicians, writers, personal assistants, etc., associated with them to be unemployed.

2.1 Research Efforts Directed to Study the Varied Dimensions Estimating the Impact of COVID-19 on Gig Economy

As of today, there is no official, fool-proof data available on the number of people working in the gig economy the world over, their characteristics, and the kind of work they are engaged in. There is not enough information for developing estimates of the impact made by COVID-19 in a global gig economy. However, efforts have been made in these gig-economy-related domains by a few erudite and expert economists and some renowned research institutes. A few of such findings and observations obtained from their work are presented below.

- Employment may increase following the recession in the gig economy. It is referred to as recession-push self-employment rather than being unemployed (Congregado et al. 2012).

- Employers also switch to using more insecure forms of work and uncertainty rises, such as temporary agency work. (Houseman and Heinrich 2015).

- The research conducted to learn the short-term effects of the pandemic in the UK, it was found that self-employed have suffered more in terms of a decline in hours and earnings in March 2020 as compared to regular employees (Adams-Prassl et al. 2020; Blundelland Machin, Blundell, and Machin 2020).

- A project at the Oxford Martin School investigating the effect of new technology on the labor market, including the gig economy (*The Future of Work*, https://www.oxfordmartin.ox.ac.uk/future-of-work).

- Oxford University is developing a new index measuring supply and demand for online freelance labor in real-time (*iLabour Project*, https://ilabour.oii. ox.ac.uk/).

- A Turing Institute project is investigating the preferences and constraints of gig-economy workers (*Labor Supply in the Gig Economy*). The authors (Muhammad Umar et al. 2020) in their paper studying the impact of COVID-19 on the gig economy have used the Online Labor Index of Oxford University as a measure of gig economy. They have used the daily record of new cases and deaths of corona patients as praxis of COVID-19. Their findings show that the pandemic has a significant positive impact on new job openings and the online job filling affected the spread the spread of the pandemic.

Abi Adams-Passl of University of Oxford; Diane Covle from the University of Cambridge; Nikhil Datta from Centre for Economic Performance, LSE; Carl Benedickt Frey from Oxford Martin School; Giulia Giupponi from Institute of Fiscal Studies; and StefenMachin from Centre for Economic Performance, LSE are some of the UK experts currently engaged in the research work related to studying the impact of the pandemic on the gig economy.

2.2. Global Scenario of Gig Economy during Pandemic

With the onset of COVID-19, the number of gig workers the world over has spiraled. According to the study conducted by

ADP Research Institute (*2021 Market Share and Data Analysis*), the gig economy accounts for a third of the world's working population expected to cross the $500 billion mark in gross volume within a five-year period. Let us have a look at the general gig economy statistics, the demographics of gig economy workers, the impact of COVID-19 on the gig economy, etc.

- Gig economy has the second-highest number of work opportunities offered. Twenty-four percent of workers across 19 countries are full-time gig workers while 9% are also employed in a traditional setting. Professional services account for most of the part-time (14.9%) and full-time (17%) gig workers. (Hayes et al. 2019)

- Approximately 68 million workers in the United States work freelance. By 2028, the population of US-based freelance workers is projected to reach 90.1 million (Keerlery 2021).

- 75% of freelancers work in the arts and design industry compared to only 25% of non-freelancers (Upwork 2020).

- 78% of gig workers plan to do the same gig work or more in the next year. Forty percent of workers participate in gig work while still employed, compared to 30% who prefer doing only gig work full time (DaVinci Payments 2021).

- 58% of the gig economy's billion-dollar gross volume is generated from transportation-based services like ridesharing and carpooling platforms. (Mastercard and Kaiser Associates 2019)

2.3 Demographics of Gig Economy Workers

The following statistics describe the demographic profiles of gig workers.

- 59% of freelancers in the US are male and 40% are female. (Keerley 2019)

Fifty-three percent of the freelancers' population in the US are made up of Gen Zers or those aged 18–22 years old (Upwork 2019). In 2020, 26% of freelancers were 55 years old and older. Sixty-five percent of freelancers in the 50-year-old and older age bracket, see freelancing as an ideal transition into retirement. Fifty percent of Gen Zers have participated in freelance work in the past 12 months (Upwork 2020; *Freelance Foreword* 2020).

2.3.1 Gig Economy Workers' Income Statistics

- Gig economy wages and participation grew 33% in 2020. The estimated total earnings of adult US-based gig economy workers was $1.6 trillion in 2020.70% of gig economy workers admit that they would be more loyal to a gig work that pays them on the same day. Of gig workers, 72% would like relevant special savings offers delivered with their gig work pay. More than 50% of independent workers from different parts of the world are supplemental earners. An additional 61% of gig workers believe it is important to use scheduling tools for tracking work hours (DaVinci Payments 2021).

- Approximately 48% of freelancers prefer to get paid based on their fixed rate, while 29% prefer an hourly rate.

- More than 50% of gig workers are GenZers and millennials who have an annual household income of $50,000 or less (Statista Research Department 2021)

- An hourly rate of gig workers in the US can range between $31–$115 (Sbai 2021)

- Nearly 17.8% of part-time gig workers participate in the gig economy for additional income (Hayes et al. 2019).

3.0 Negative Impact of COVID-19 on Existing Freelancers

The studies referred to in sections 4.1 and 4.2 suggest the pandemic has spiraled the growth of the gig economy. However, a negative impact of the pandemic on existing freelancers is observed in the study conducted by Upwork in 2020. The following findings of the said study unveil this fact.

- Approximately 10% of US-based freelancers have paused freelancing at the onset of COVID-19.

- Approximately 28% of paused freelancers are either on leave or unemployed, and 51% still have other sources of work.

- Approximately 41% of freelancers have been doing less work during the pandemic.

- Approximately 17% of paused freelancers are made up of students, homemakers, and retirees.

- Among the paused freelancers, 88% are still willing to do freelance work in the future.

Traditional labor markets the world over, having been hit hard by COVID-19, freelancing, and remote work which were previously overshadowed by traditional office jobs are perceived as new trends reshaping future employment and business operations. The regular workers, who now feel comfortable with a work-from-home model, indicate it would be difficult for them to go back to the original 9–5 or 10–6 work schedule even after the pandemic.

3.1 Some Observations about Impact of COVID-19 on Gig/Sharing Economy

The report published by OECD (2021) which studied in depth the impact of the growth of the sharing and gig economy on VAT/GST policy and administration contained the following observations with regard to the impact of COVID-19 on gig/sharing economy:

- It has impacted activity in the two largest sectors of the gig economy (i.e., the sectors of transportation [ride-sourcing] and of short-term accommodation [real estate rental]).

- It is likely to have a positive impact on certain types of gig/sharing activity, such as online teaching, delivery of food and other items sold online, short-term rental of online working space, etc.

- To some extent, the platforms that generate and facilitate gig/sharing economy activity may be in a better position to weather the COVID-19 crisis than their competitors in the traditional industries as they have more flexibility in managing their costs and risks. This may apply to the larger gig economy platform operators that have continual access to finance.

- Some smaller gig/sharing economy platforms during the crisis became a lifeline for traditional businesses in certain sectors like restaurants, adapting to new ways of serving their customers.

These businesses would, in all likelihood, continue using the new, technology-based distribution even after the crisis.

- It could be expected that more and more people continue to supplement their income even after the crisis by monetizing their skills and assets via the gig economy.

- Also, it could be expected that several new habits developed during the pandemic may continue even after the crisis. For example, the live-and-work anywhere mindset that has grown up during the pandemic may lead to an increase in demand in the rental of short-term accommodation.

3.2 The BCG and Michael and Susan Dell Foundation Report

The recent report jointly published by the global management consulting firm Boston Consulting Group (BCG) and the nonprofit organization Michael & Susan Dell Foundation maintained gig work has gained momentum in recent years due to the emergence and success of platform-based firms such as Uber, Swiggy, Zomato, and Urban Company. The report further argued participation in the gig economy is more in developing countries (between 5% and 12%) than in developed countries (between 1% and 4%), and most of the jobs are in lower-income job types such as deliveries, ridesharing, micro-tasks, care, and wellness.

Most of the affected countries undertook several measures like lockdowns, business shutdowns, hygiene regulations, schools and universities closing, or mobility tracing to slow down the spread of COVID-19 (Spark and Straub 2020). The authors focused on the flexible employment relationship that includes gig workers also and careers in the times of the COVID-19 pandemic. They wanted to find out how the work and careers of individuals in flexible employment relationships might get affected.

The specific COVID-19 related challenges of three gig-work populations; rideshare and delivery drivers; hairstylists, barbers and aestheticians, and sex workers are discussed by Jean (2020).

The global labor studies are analyzed (Maria et al. 2020) and the authors have addressed many pertinent questions whose rational answers may help build up an emerging agenda for the global gig economy. The questions are like how the pandemic is reconfiguring the global and national, how is the destabilizing distinction between formal and informal sectors, how did it exacerbate inequalities and sharpen the class divide, what would be the consequences for workers, would there be significant potential shifts and realignments as a result of the pandemic, what about the global ecological crisis, etc.

It is evident from real-time surveys analyzed (Adams and Prassl 2020) that different countries are impacted differently. Germany has been relatively less affected by the crisis than in US and UK. Employees with temporary contracts have been more likely to lose their jobs.

4.0 International Gig Economy Scenario

4.1 Impact of the Pandemic on US Gig Economy

The gig economy has remained an integral part of the US economy that trend is accelerated during COVID-19. It has grossly affected the conventional 9–5 work in the offices and has caused many blue- and white-collar employees to turn to gig work for supplemental or even primary income.

Some pre-COVID-19 estimates predict that roughly 57 million Americans are currently engaged in some type of gig work that contributes more than $1 trillion to the US economy annually. But the post-COVID-19 scenario of the US gig economy would be altogether different.

Rebbeca Henderson, the executive board member of Randstad and CEO of the company's global businesses, described the kind of changes in the US gig economy caused by COVID-19, how COVID-19 has transformed the gig economy

- According to her, 70% of gig workers participated out of choice before the pandemic, it is likely that many full-time employees have had to reluctantly do the gig work out of necessity. The advantage of flexibility in gig work is always welcomed, but the COVID-19-pushed flexibility may not pay off favorably.

- Working parents have been forced to play a dual role as work-from-home employees and homeschool teachers as many offices and schools have closed their physical doors.

- Since the start of the pandemic, the demand for gig workers has spiraled, the competition for gig jobs has also increased. Workers who participate in the gig economy as their sole source of income must now compete with one another, as well as previously full-time employees who have been pushed into gig work. Some businesses may derive a cost advantage from such a scenario; workers themselves will have to establish their personal brands by widening their skill sets.

- The gig workers benefit from flexibility but are devoid of the benefits of health insurance. The debate in the corporate world during COVID-19 continues around these two crucial issues as to how to strike balance between the two. The Prop 22 vote in California, a measure that allowed businesses to classify gig workers as independent contractors but required them to provide them with a healthcare contribution subsidy and 120% of the local minimum wages. Such provision calls for collaboration among employers, workers, and state governments.

- In the wake of the availability of several vaccines now, the pandemic hopefully may weaken or vanish in the days to come, and the world economies might tend to turn to normalcy. The businesses will have to relook at and reevaluate the role the gig workers play in the organization and work out a plan to retain them.

A Gallup study by McFeely and Pandell (2020) found that 36% of the US labor force (57 million people) are gig workers. According to the study from Lyft drivers to sex workers, gig work involves a formal or informal contract between a company or a person compensates the laborer in a typically monetary form. COVID-19 gives an opportunity to policymakers to redefine the classification of labor.

4.2 Impact of the Pandemic on the Canadian Gig Economy

There is a peculiar situation in Canada regarding tracking the gig economy and gig workers due to the lack of necessary up-to-date data. Despite the significant share of gig workers in the Canadian labor force, it is more difficult again to measure the impact of the pandemic on the Canadian gig economy as here gig workers enter various nonstandard work arrangements to complete specific tasks or work for a specific period. Their work-loss is therefore not captured by standard employment or wage indicators.

One study (Jeon et al. 2019) has brought out several important aspects of the Canadian gig economy. They have tried to describe the demographic profile of the gig workers, the place of their residence, and the industry of their work. The study also tried to find out who would be eligible for governmental benefits.

According to this study, 19% of male gig workers and 17% of female gig workers provided professional and technical services (figure 1). In contrast, the gig workers in arts and entertainment (8.2% of male and 7.2% of female gig workers) may find it difficult to continue their business activities as social distancing is likely to remain in place for a pretty long period. Gig workers, especially in service industries, would have a comparatively harder time dealing with the economic fall out of the pandemic as in these industries necessitate face-to-face interaction with customers. In the transportation industry, where there are male gig workers (8.3% of total) and are mostly the Uber and Lyft partners, it would be difficult for them to continue their work either because these companies may curtail their operations or because of the reduction in the number of riders.

Similarly, the female gig workers in the industries such as retail with 10% of female gig workers in it, administrative and support services like tour operators, cleaning service providers (13.4 % of female gig workers), and other services like cooks. Maids, nannies (12.7% of total female gig workers) would have a difficult period ahead and may have to suffer huge employment losses (Statistics, Canada 2020).

Chart 1
Industrial distribution of gig workers

Industry

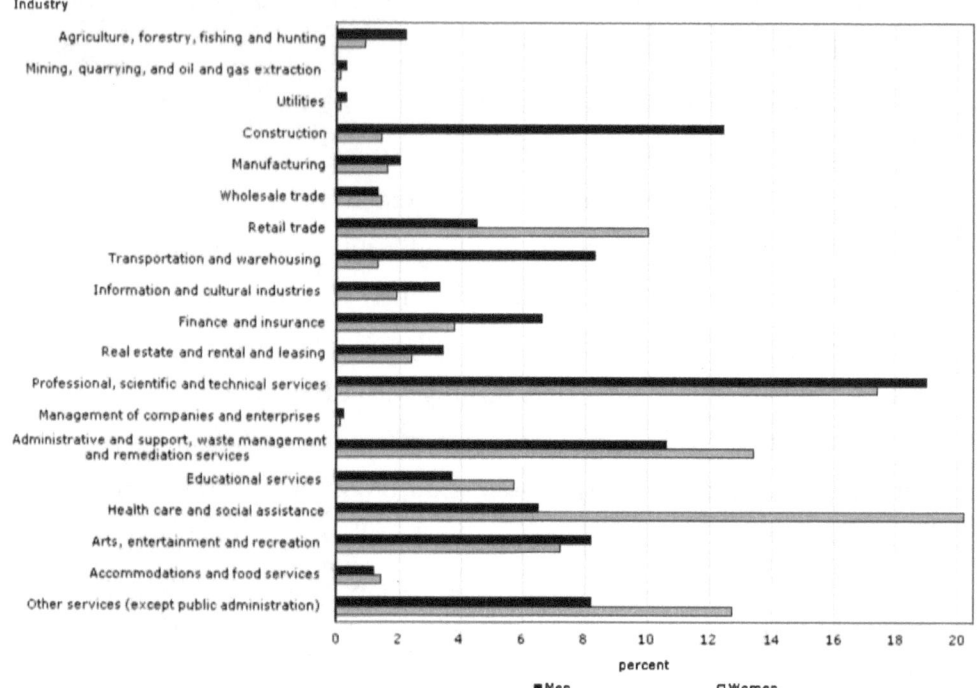

Note: Based on Table 3 in Jeon et al. (2019).
Source: Statistics Canada.

The study also probed into the questions related to how the gig economy would evolve in the aftermath of the COVID-19. According to the study, the size of the gig economy increased from 6% in 2008 to 6.8% in 2009 as some of those who lost their wage employment during the recession were *pushed* into self-employment. Whether a similar trend will occur in the aftermath of COVID-19 will likely depend on the speed and intensity of the post-COVID-19 overall economic recovery. Another important question is whether the current pandemic will facilitate the expansion of online platforms potentially leading to the increase in the size of the gig economy. The real challenge for the researchers in the forthcoming period is to continue to improve the methodology and timeliness of measuring the gig economy in Canada and assessing the financial condition of gig workers and their families.

4.3 Impact of the Pandemic on Brazil Gig Economy

Brazil is among the countries which are worst hit by the pandemic. The first case of COVID-19 in Brazil was announced by the Ministry of Health on February 26, 2020. Two weeks earlier, the Brazilian Institute of Geography and Statistics (IGBE) had published data from the National Household Survey showing that around 38 million people in Brazil work in the informal sector. In eleven out of 27 states, more than 50% of workers were in the informal sector and therefore fell outside the bounds of protective labor laws. Beyond informal work, a recent report by researchers from Rede de Pesquisa Solidaria estimated that the pandemic would hit up to 81% of the country's labor force, thereby impacting even supposedly secure jobs.

Brazil is the seventh most unequal country in the world in terms of income distribution. The same inequality is surfaced in the country's heterogeneous labor market that is mostly stratified by race and gender. Across the labor force as a whole, the average monthly income of the white population ($486) was 74% higher than that of the black and brown population ($279). Accordingly, vulnerability is higher amongst black and brown people (Tamb'em dispon'ivel em portugues). Since the beginning of the health crisis, Brazil's president Jair Bolsonaro was not at all in favor of the complete lockdown that was fully resisted by public health experts. But somehow the move could fend off a further recession for a while. But in the month of March 2021, the infected cases again started surging with a new record high of 1,641 deaths on a particular day. That caused a further economic slowdown.

The state-run Fiocruz Institute said that that ICU occupation rates in 18 states and the Federal District had surpassed 80%—a level considered to be critical.

Many state governors, scientists, mayors, and health experts have been insisting on tighter restrictions and President Bolsonaro continued opposing them. But according to the last year's verdict of the Supreme Court of Brazil, such decisions are local authorities' prerogative.

There is a silver lining amid the dark and dense clouds of deaths and devastation caused by the pandemic. According to IGBE data, Brazil saw a robust rebound in the back half of 2020 with 7.7% and 3.2% growth in the third and fourth quarters. Family consumption went up in both quarters supported by the government welfare program though the phenomenon was observed to be short-lived. As mass vaccination progresses, it is expected by the economists that the services industry of Brazil that is badly hit by the pandemic may start recovering by the second half of next year. Goldman Sach's chief Latin America economist Alberto Ramos, talking about Brazil's service industry plight, said, "In the very near term, the recent pick up in new viral cases, the acceleration of inflation and the phasing out of some of the generous fiscal transfer programs may soften the momentum behind the recovery of service sectors."

The fate of Brazil's creative workers in the gig economy during this turbulent time was at stake. They were living on the edge (Diego and Vieira 2021). According to the authors, they were open to exploitation, getting lower wages, and having a lower level of satisfaction during the pandemic as compared to earlier. They become even more exposed to the lack of long-standing protections, such as minimum wage, safety, and health regulation, retirement income, health insurance, and worker compensation. Now they are also exposed to risks that were formerly shouldered by employers and the state including responsibility for bodily injury, damage to tools and assets, coverage between paid gigs, financial malfeasance by customers, and harassment.

Narrating the plight of food delivery workers and their collective organization in Brazil based on social media (Helena et al.), the authors say that the COVID-19 pandemic exacerbated and increased the visibility of the precarious work conditions experienced by those who use digital platforms in Rio de Janeiro, Brazil. Now they are collectively organized throughout Brazil to demand better work conditions. In July 2020, there were two national strikes by them to demonstrate their protest.

4.4 The Impact of COVID-19 on the Indian Gig Economy

India had a large informal sector for several years which was a major source of employment for casual workers. What has changed in recent years is the infusion of technology into these on-demand services. The Boston Consulting Group (BCG) report argues that in the next three to four years, India's gig economy would triple and might create around 90 million jobs in the next 8–10 years. For the same time period, it could transact over $ 250 billion worth of work in terms of volume and subsequently, contribute at least 1.25% to India's GDP in the long term. The report highlights four sectors which are responsible for such a rise in the gig economy: manufacturing, construction, retail, transportation, and logistics.

It is interesting to research as to which are the contributing factors giving thrust to gig work. The pandemic-induced uncertainty is, of course, one of the key reasons. But according to the experts, the growth in the gig economy can also be attributed to both demand and supply-related factors in the wake of pandemic-induced uncertainty. But the demand push from the organization side depicts only half of the picture. India's demographic dividend—the young and energetic youths have different perceptions and expectations with regard to the concepts of work-life balance, happiness, etc. A gig economy provides them the flexibility to decide what one wants to do (or not to do), when, for whom, and from where.

A similar view is expressed in the report (January 2021) by the industry body Association of Indian Chambers of Commerce (Assocham). It reads, "With talent pools today becoming way more diverse in their age constitution and with millennials and Gen Z workers increasingly becoming the part of the country's workforce, may have begun preferring to become part of the gig economy."

It further says, "As more and more companies undertake business transformation to make their processes more technology-driven, the number of gig workers are bound to go up. Increasing use of technology, like AI and automation, would also lead to the creation of new job profiles and a business's need to look for qualified talent. In the coming years, instead of hiring outright for such positions, it would be possible for companies to just reach out to talent on a more project-like basis."

A Flourish Venture survey (2020) highlighted that "90% of Indian gig workers lost their income during the pandemic. They earned more than Rs. 25000 per month before the pandemic. By August 2020, 9 in 10 were earning less than Rs. 15,000 per month and more than 33.3% were earning Rs.150 per day or less."

Due to this lost income, many workers were forced to take a drastic step to make ends meet such as 44% borrowed, 45% reduced their essential expenditures, and 83% used their savings. According to the survey, "India stands to lose 135 million jobs because of the pandemic and this is likely to push the full-time workforce toward the gig economy. Moreover, many laid-off employees are focusing on developing skills to avail freelance job opportunities and become a part of this burgeoning economy."

The case of ride-hailing companies was studied (Sabrina Korrack 2020). According to it, in the ride-hailing sector, drivers have lost substantial amounts of their incomes, which implies that many of them are struggling to cover their essential needs, let alone pay financial obligations from financing, leasing, or renting the cars that they use for their gigs. In addition, drivers are exposed to a risk of infection with the SARS-COV-2, and if they are infected, they face off financial pressure to continue to work and might end up endangering themselves and their passengers and further contributing to the spread of the virus. Uber and Ola have responded with several measures. Overall, the finding of the study suggests that COVID-19-related measures are more appearance than substance and provide neither sufficient health protection nor adequate financial support.

In one more study on gig work and platforms during the COVID-19 in India (Shipra Minaketan 2020), the author has highlighted major dilemmas faced by the service providers during the full and partial lockdown. Uber and Ola drivers who have to pay EMIs for their cars have complained about not getting enough work to even justify the cost of sanitizers and petrol they are spending on.

4.5 Impact of COVID-19 on Gig Economy of UK

The "Gig Economy Statistics, UK, Industry Report, 2021" provides the following valuable statistics of the UK gig economy:

- 1 in 7 adults in the UK has done a gig job monthly.
- Gig workers contribute 20 billion pounds to the UK economy the same as the aerospace industry.

- 48% of gig workers in the UK also have full-time jobs.

- Women earn an average of 10% less than males in the gig economy.

- For most, 71.5% of gig work makes up less than half of their income.

- 7.25 million people are likely to work in the gig economy in 2022.

The latest official figures show that Britain's gig economy sat at 4.7 million people in 2019, more than double the size of 2.4 million from 2016. At this time, it is around 9.6% of the working population who are delivering gig work at least once a month.

Gig-based freelancers contribute approximately 20 billion pounds to the British economy each year according to the report of Centre for Research and Self-Employment (Center for Research and Self-Employment 2019, *The Freelance Project and Gig Economies of the 21ˢᵗ Century*, https://crse.co.uk/research/freelance HYPERLINK "https://crse.co.uk/research/freelance–project-and-gig-economies-21ˢᵗ–century"– HYPERLINK "https://crse.co.uk/research/freelance–project-and-gig-economies-21ˢᵗ–century"project-and-gig-economies- HYPERLINK "https://crse.co.uk/research/freelance–project-and-gig-economies-21ˢᵗ–century"21 HYPERLINK "https://crse.co.uk/research/freelance–project-and-gig-economies-21ˢᵗ–century"st HYPERLINK "https://crse.co.uk/research/freelance–project-and-gig-economies-21ˢᵗ–century"– HYPERLINK "https://crse.co.uk/research/freelance–project-and-gig-economies-21ˢᵗ–century"century).

The report estimates that 3.2 billion pounds (16%) of the British economy contribution is made of earnings from Uber drivers

("Uber: The Impact of Uber in the UK," https://www.uber.com/en-GB/ newsroom/the impact-of-uber-in-the-uk) while one study by Capital Economics (Deliverloo, "Deliverloo Will Create 70,000 Jobs," https:// uk.deliverloo.news/creating-restaurants-jobs-html) believes Deliverloo would contribute 1.5 billion pounds to the British economy.

4.5.1 Popular Gig Economy Platforms in the UK

The gig economy platforms that have become popular in the UK include Uber, Deliverloo, PeoplePerHour, Fiverr, Upwork, TaskRabbit, AmazonFlex, etc.

4.5.2 Demographics of Gig Workers in the UK

An estimated 16.5% of the UK male population is involved in the gig economy, 14% of the UK female population is engaged in gig works. Among all gig workers, women occupy around 46.5%.

As per their age distribution, 35% of the gig workforce belong to the 16–24 years age group, 16.4% belong to the age group of 25–34 years whereas 13.4% belong to the age group of 45–54 years.

Women earn an average of 10% less than men in the gig economy.

4.5.3 Who Was Impacted by the COVID-19 and How Much Was It in the UK Gig Economy?

Different gig works were impacted differently by COVID-19. The food-providing gig companies such as Uber Eats and Deliverloo exceeded targets during the pandemic, experiencing record-high growth in demand) due to the loss of in-person hospitality. After the first UK lockdown, Deliverloo signed up 11,500 new restaurants and announced recruitment plans for 15,000 additional drivers (6). In the middle of the pandemic (August 2020), 28% of delivery drivers reported having more work than usual.

Other types of gig-economy work such as taxi rides were heavily impacted. Uber recorded a 73% drop in the number of rides as compared with the same period last year before the pandemic has started. This would mean an average pay loss of 21,531 pounds for each Uber driver.

So far as the interest for the gig economy is concerned, the pandemic caused an increase in it to a marked extent. Ninety-two percent of respondents in the survey by the jobs board, Monster said that they think now is a good time to look into the gig economy. Just over half of people (57%) said that the gig work would be essential while they are searching for jobs during the COVID-19.

As a result of the virus, it is also expected that many companies are likely to turn to gig works in their attempt to cut costs, fueling the growth of the gig economy.

4.5.4 Advantages and Disadvantages Experienced by UK Gig Workers during the Pandemic

A pertinent question could be raised as to whether the UK gig workers benefitted from this turbulent time of the pandemic, or they were at disadvantage. One major study by the government of the UK (7) indicates that more than half (53%) of those involved in the British gig economy are either mostly or moderately satisfied with their experience of providing services in websites and apps. Ninety-four percent of gig workers who work full-time are satisfied with their employment situation.

In the said study it was observed that the following percentage of them found the pandemic advantageous:

Providing independence (58%), flexibility (56%), availability of the number of hours (46%), cost of providing services (38%), whereas the following percentage of them found this period to their disadvantage with regard to income levels (25%), work benefits (25%), career development opportunities (23%), irregular workload (18%).

According to the study, 69% were satisfied with providing courier services, 68% were happy with their taxi work, and 65% were comfortable with their job as food deliverers.

The study maintains that the UK gig economy is here to stay. One additional study by AON 2020, predicted that 18% of human resource directors in the UK think that gig workers will make up 75% or more of their workforce over the next five years.

In the UK the government prioritized large corporations and financial institutions followed by profitable businesses with three years account. The self-employed people working in the gig economy, alongside others managing zero-hour contacts, found themselves at the back of the queue. Such people have been largely abandoned by the state being left to their own devices, having to fend for themselves (Ben Duke 2020).

5.0 Measures Taken

There is hardly any country in the world that may have remained uncontaminated by the coronavirus. The overall global economy was hit hard by COVID-19. The gig economies in different countries, as we saw in earlier sections, had different impacts on the pandemic. Every country was in action mode and was trying to fight it, tooth and nail. All welfare states devised measures to protect their gig economy sector along with all other sectors of their respective economy.

Governments across OECD (Organization for Economic Co-operation and Development) countries have taken unprecedented steps to protect the self-employed by providing cash payments to the entire population, expanding access, in many cases for a short period, to sickness benefits and special paid care leave, unemployment benefits and short-term work schemes to the self-employed (OECD 2020). Fairwork Foundation survey (Fairwork 2020) of gig-economy platform policies, covering 120 platforms in 23 countries across Europe, North America, South America, Asia, and Africa has examined the platforms in the five different contexts: fair pay, fair conditions, fair contacts, fair management, and fair representations.

5.1 Measures Taken by the US

The US federal government under CARES Act (Coronavirus Aid, Relief and Economic Security Act), approved of $ 2 trillion federal stimulus package, which is considered to be an economic lifeline for gig workers and freelancers. For the first time, freelancers/gig workers are offered unemployment insurance of an additional $600 per week. Once state benefits are added to it, the weekly payouts are around $800–$900 per week.

The stimulus package also offers self-employed and small business owners a non-refundable $10,000 advance as an Emergency Economic Injury Disaster Loan (EIDL). The bill authorizes $10 billion in the appropriation for these loans. In addition, the Freelancers Union introduced Freelancers Relief Fund that offers a $1,000 emergency grant to them for necessities like rent and groceries.

In California, Proposition 22 (of course opposed by President Biden) sought to exempt Uber, Lift, Door Dash, and other firms from Assembly Bill 5, and allowed to classify gig workers as regular employees and grant them relevant benefits.

5.2 Measures Taken by Canada

The Canadian government introduced COVID-19 Emergency Response Act No. 2, to support Canadians and businesses facing troubles. The government deferred all GST/HST (Harmonized Sales Tax) payments. Business Development Bank of Canada launched the new small- and medium-sized enterprise loan and guarantee program to help weather the impact of COVID-19. Gig workers are considered to be dependent contractors, and now they have the right to unionize under labor laws. In the context of COVID-19, the substantial contribution of gig workers to the Canadian economy is now increasingly recognized. Recent legal trends seem to treat the gig workers as regular employees. The report of the Expert Panel on Modern Federal Labor Standards by Employment and Social Development Data, Canada(ESDC 2019) demonstrates the express need for and potential advantages of securing stronger protection for gig workers.

5.3 Measures Taken by Brazil

Brazil's congress has approved of an $8 billion emergency aid package to help deal with the second wave of the pandemic that had triggered economic shutdown across the country. Though the amount is not enough to meet with the disaster created by the pandemic, it may prevent at least the people from going hungry. Also, they have announced a cash transfer scheme providing $40 per month to the nation's poorest for the next couple of months.

5.4 Measures Taken by the Indian Government

To provide aid and support to these gig workers, the Indian government has undertaken several measures. "The Code on Social

Security" passed by the government would provide the workers with life and disability cover. Accidental insurance, health and maternity benefits, old age protection, etc. Under the code, the central and state governments will primarily fund social security measures with a nominal contribution (1%–2% of their annual turnover) by the aggregator. Also, the contribution made by the aggregator/platform will not exceed 5% of the amount payable to gig and platform workers. In addition, the code proposed to establish a National Social Security Board which will supervise and formulate schemes for the well-being of gig and platform workers.

The gig economy has been on the rise in India. During the pandemic more and more gig workers are transitioning from full-time employment. The government can offer them mandatory coverage under existing schemes like Bharat Pradhan Mantri Jan Arogya Yojana, Pradhan Mantri Suraksha Vima Yojana, Pradhan Mantri Jeevan Jyoti Bima Yojana, etc.

5.5 Measures Taken by the UK

The UK government announced a package of 30 billion pounds what the finance minister Rishi Sunak described as "one of the most generous support programs" anywhere in the world. The program provides Britain's 5 million self-employed workers a cash grant of 80% of their average monthly profit up to 2,500 pounds a month over the next quarter. He also announced a 500-million pound boost to help those who could not work during the pandemic. It includes statutory sick pay for all people who are isolated from the virus, earlier benefits payments for the self-employed, and the removal of the minimum income floor from Universal Credit. The UK government made a provision of a 1.2 million pounds interruption loan for small and medium-sized businesses affected by COVID-19.

UK's fine-tech communication has built Covid Credit to let sole traders self-certify lost income. It is envisaged that government relief extended to salaried workers might now be extended to self-employed gig workers through open banking technology.

6.0 Conclusions

The COVID-19 pandemic has triggered the deepest economic recession world over, threatening health, disrupting economic activities, hurting the well-being, and cruelly snatching away millions of lives and jobs. Globally, the pandemic has highlighted the sheer level of precarity engendered by the global restructuring of labor markets. The pandemic has hit hard the countries across the globe, regardless of the fact that it may be developed, developing, or underdeveloped country. The gig economy of every country also had to bear the brunt due to the disaster of such magnitude that creates horrors once in a century. Millions of people with no full-time jobs or whose businesses rely on people getting together such as taxi drivers, food deliverers, hairdressers, gym and spa owners, etc., were rendered helpless as governments announced a shutdown of nonessential services and introduced strict social distancing measures. Though most of the gig economies of the world received the death blow, a few of them were found thriving during such turbulent times in some countries.

Extraordinary policies were required to walk the tight rope toward recovery. The intelligent and farsighted moves were needed in formulating the stimulus packages and relief measures to revive the gig economies and shape the social prospects. Critically analyzing the measures adopted by different countries, it is observed that they do not substantially provide for gig workers. At the same time, measures announced by on-demand service companies are inadequate, ambiguous, and inconsistent. The eligibility, process, and quantum of relief are unclear to them.

Several countries have adopted emergency transfer programs that target vulnerable groups stirring up the debates around universal basic income as a mechanism that can redistribute wealth and expand ingress to citizenship.

The efforts need to be combined involving federal/state governments with on-demand service companies. While preparing the stimulus package, it should be done in collaboration with the gig workers. The efforts with regard to their healthcare protection, socioeconomic protection, effective communication of such measures, etc., should be bolstered.

Minimum wage rates defined for skilled workers in the respective state/country should be paid to the gig workers too. All healthcare-related schemes/benefits could be extended to the gig workers. Medical insurances, if provided to the gig workers may prove to be a boon to them in such a horrible time. Personal protection equipment should be provided to them free of cost.

The interests on the different loans borrowed by them should generously be forgiven for some well-defined period. All granular and regular information regarding the relief measures should be regularly communicated to them. Assurance should be given to them that once the pandemic is over, they would be back to their gig work as earlier.

References

Adams-Prassl, Abi, Rauh, Chrostopher. 2020. "Inequality in the impact of coronavirus shock: Evidence from real-time surveys." *Journal of Public Economics*, vol. 189, 104245.

Behera, Shipra Mineketan. 2020. "Gig Work and Platforms during the COVID-19 Pandemic in India." *Engage*, vol.55, issue no. 45.

Benjamin, Duke. 2020. "The effects of the covid-19 crisis on the gig economy and zero-hour contacts," *Interface: A journal for and about social movements*, Group 24, 8.

Congregado, E., Golpe, A., van Stel, A. 2012. "The 'recession-push' hypothesis reconsidered." *International Entrepreneurship and Management Journal*, 8, 325–342. https://doi.org/ HYPERLINK "https://doi.org/10.1007/s11365-011-0176-1"10.1007 HYPERLINK "https://doi.org/10.1007/s11365-011-0176-1"/s HYPERLINK "https://doi.org/10.1007/s11365-011-0176-1"11365-011-0176-1.

daVanci Payments. 2021. "daVanci Payments study shows boom in the gig economy and how to attract gig workers and grow their loyalty." *Business Wire*. Retrieved April 15, 2021.

Department for Business, Energy, Industrial Engineering. 2018. "The characteristics of those in the Gig Economy." *Final Report*.

Fairwork. 2020. "The Gig Economy and COVID-19." *Fairwork Report on Platform Policies*. Oxford, United Kingdom. https://fair.work/fair-work-releases -report-on-platform-responses-to-covid-HYPERLINK "https://fair.work/fair-work-releases%20-report-on-platform-responses-to-covid-19/"19 HYPERLINK "https://fair.work/fair-work-releases%20-report-on-platform-responses-to-covid-19/"/

Hynes, M., Chummye, F., Wright C., and Buckingham, M. 2019. "The global study of engagement: Technical Report," ADP Research Institute.

Houseman, S. N. and Heinrich, C. J. 2015. "Temporary help employment in recession and recovery." *Upjohn Institute Working*

Papers (May 1), 15–227. https://orcid.org/ HYPERLINK "https://orcid.org/0000-0003-2657-8479"0000-0003-2657-8479.

Jeon, S. H., Liu, Huju, and Osrtovsky, Yuri. 2019. "Measuring the Gig Economy in Canada Using Administrative Data," *Analytical Studies Branch Research Paper Series*, catalog number: 11F0019M, No. 437. Ottawa Statistics, Canada.

Korak, Sabrina. 2020. "COVID-19 and India's gig economy, the case of ride-hailing companies," *ORF ISSUE BRIEF*, issue 377.

Maria Lorena Cook, Madhumitta Dutta, Alexander, Jorg, Ben Scally (2020). Global labor studies in the pandemic: Notes for an Emerging Agenda, Global Labor Journal. 11 (2), 74-83.

McFeely, S. and Pendell, R. 2020. "What Workplace Leaders Can Learn from the Real Gig Economy, Gallup?"

OECD. 2020, "Paid sick leave to protect income, health and jobs through the COVID-19 crisis." *OECD Policy Responsesto Coronavirus.* OECD Publishing, Paris.

OECD. 2021. "The impact of the Growth of the Sharing and Gig economy on VAT/GST Policy and Administration." *OECD*, ISBN: 9789264914780(PDF).

Santos, Diego, de Jesus, Vieira. 2021. *Psychology*, 11 (2): 56–62.

Sbai, A. 2021. "The gig-work platform's market sheds its skin to face COVID's impact." *Infomineo.* Retrieved April 15, 2021.

Spark, D., Straub, C. 2020. "Flexible employment relationship and careers in times of COVID-19 Pandemic." *Journal of Vocational Behavior*, vol. 119, 103435.

Statistics Canada. 2020. *Labor Force Survey, April 2020.* www.statcan. Gc.ca/n1/daily-quotidien /200508/ dq200508a-eng.htm.

Statista Research Department. 2019. *Freelance Workers by Gender, U.S. 2019* (May 11). https://www.statista.com/statistics/ HYPERLINK "https://www.statista.com/statistics/531002/freelance-workers-by-gender-us/"531002 HYPERLINK "https://www.statista.com/statistics/531002/freelance-workers-by-gender-us/"/ freelance-workers-by-gender-us/.

Statista Research Department. 2021. "Gig Economy: Number of Freelancers in the US, 2017–28." *Statista.* Retrieved April 15, 2021.

Strecker, Helena, Sampario, Ana Luiza, Buritica, Juan, Aroso, Laura, Rubin, Kavina. et al. 2021. "The Collective Organization of Delivery Workers in Brazil during the COVID-19 Pandemic: A View Based on Social Media."

Tyara, Jean. 2020. "The Gig is Up: Supporting Non-Standard Workers Now and After Coronavirus." *Learner Centre for Public Health Promotion*, issue no. 19. Syracuse University.

Umar, Muhmad, Xo, Yan, and Mirza, Sultan Sikandar N. 2020. "The Impact of COVID-19 on Gig Economy." *Economic Research— Ekonomska Instrazuvanja*, DOI: 10, 1080/1331677X, 2020, 1862680.

Upwork. 2020. *New Upwork Study Finds 36% of the U.S. Workforce Freelance Amid the COVID-19 Pandemic* (September 15). Retrieved November 28. https://www.upwork.com/press/ releases/new-upwork-study-finds- HYPERLINK "https:// www.upwork.com/press/releases/new-upwork-study-finds-36-of-the-us-workforce-freelance-amid-the-covid-19-pandemic"36 HYPERLINK "https://www.upwork.com/press/releases/new-upwork-study-finds-36-of-the-us-workforce-freelance-amid-the-covid-19-pandemic"-of-the-us-workforce-freelance-amid-the-

covid- HYPERLINK "https://www.upwork.com/press/releases/
new-upwork-study-finds-36-of-the-us-workforce-freelance-
amid-the-covid-19-pandemic"19 HYPERLINK "https://www.
upwork.com/press/releases/new-upwork-study-finds-36-of-the-
us-workforce-freelance-amid-the-covid-19-pandemic"-pandemic

CHAPTER 4

Economic Impact of a Pandemic: Survival and Recovery

by Toni McIntosh

Abstract

The impact of a pandemic can cripple a relatively unstable economy. The impact on the United States economy, including the stock market, is incomparable to any global pandemic in history. A strong economy is less likely to sustain a substantial hit; however, the severity and duration of the COVID-19 pandemic tested the strength of even the strongest economy. History shows that in the four recorded pandemics over the last 131 years, an understanding of viral infections, and their spread is vital to successfully address the overall impact of the health crisis. A halt on in-person learning, dining, shopping, and state-mandated curfews in the early months of the COVID-19 pandemic created hardship for individuals, families, and businesses. Business owners quickly learned that their current processes would no longer sustain them, presenting an opportunity to review and change how they operated to maintain revenue.

Unemployment rates skyrocketed to 14.8 percent in the early months of the pandemic as a result of businesses closing indefinitely. A push to reopen states in order to stimulate the economy has exhausted attempts to slow the spread of the virus, and businesses are forced to change their processes in order to reenter the economy and stay afloat. Leaders and managers are faced with revamping office space to accommodate returning employees while significant losses and slow rebounds still plague the markets as the world seeks to recover from a globally devastating health crisis.

Keywords: COVID-19, economic losses, shutdowns, pandemic, stock market, unemployment, process change

1.0 Introduction

On January 9, 2020, the World Health Organization (WHO), in response to reports from Chinese officials, reported that the recent outbreak in Wuhan, China, initially dubbed pneumonia cases, was indeed an outbreak of a novel coronavirus (World Health Organization 2020). Between January and March 2020, the virus spread across the globe. Asia, Europe, and the United States scrambled to prepare to combat this highly contagious and quick-spreading disease (Baccini and Brodeur 2021). Strict handwashing, social distancing, and mask-wearing mandates were instituted across the United States. Citizens were advised to shelter in place to reduce the spread of the virus as government officials in individual states within the country took matters into their own hands by establishing curfews and mandating the closure of nonessential businesses (Thorbecke 2020). The world and its citizens were faced with establishing a new normal when the global pandemic disrupted life. In the months to come, the virus claimed hundreds of thousands of lives globally and caused tremendous economic damage to the countries in its path. The damage sustained by the economy was likened to consequences experienced during the 2008 global financial crisis (Baccini and Brodeur 2021).

1.1 The Early Days of the Pandemic

At the beginning of the pandemic, decisions were made to address halting the spread of the virus. The most prominent action available at the time was to lockdown the affected countries since there was no vaccine to combat the virus (Baccini and Brodeur, 2021). Amid the shutdown, restaurants were confined to takeout orders only with no indoor dining. Masked patrons placed to-go orders and had them delivered to their homes or picked up outside the restaurant. Businesses closed their doors and sent nonessential employees home to work remotely. Information technology was in overdrive as virtual private networks (VPNs) and remote connectivity sessions tested the strength of an organization's technology infrastructure. Zoom cloud meetings, though in existence for several years, became the go-to for remote meetings by business organizations and families to keep in touch. Likewise, social media usage increased as individuals used these outlets to share information and keep in touch with others.

As time passed, several societal components of the pandemic were identified as highly impactful both negatively and positively to the economy.

- Mandatory shelter-in-place orders: Cities, states, and eventually entire countries made the decision to require their citizens to remain at home and limit contact with others outside their household. The effects of the shelter-in-place orders proved to be commensurable to those in the shutdowns (Asahi et al. 2021).

- Increased demand for telecommunication devices and services to aid in maintaining a sense of normalcy to daily living, individuals craved a means of not only checking on their loved ones since visitations were on hold but also the need to maintain communication with coworkers, friends, and peers.

- A decrease in an active workforce: The fear of contracting the virus in a germ-infested workplace caused some workers to quit their jobs. Others worked for industries that shut down during the pandemic as they experienced a drastic decline in business, or the business was deemed nonessential.

- There is an enormous increase in the need for healthcare, hospitalizations, and burial services as the virus quickly spread across the country, and indeed, the globe, the need for immediate health care rose dramatically with hospitals overrun with COVID-19 cases. Clinical providers, quite possibly deemed the most critical essential workers, worked long shifts to care for the droves of individuals flooding hospital emergency rooms. Sadly, families were also faced with quickly obtaining burial services for their loved ones who rapidly succumbed to the virus, creating an increase in the need for funeral and mortuary services.

- A stagnated reopening process for states and businesses: Amid a flurry of public demand and rallying, some local governments were cautious in approaching a reopening to business as usual. In some cases, the increase in positive COVID-19 cases was not a deterrent for those individuals and groups (parents of school children, primarily) who insisted that the government remove mandated closings of businesses, schools, and entertainment facilities (Walmsley and Wei 2021).

Panic buying by consumers early in the pandemic produced a sense of fear and uncertainty as buyers emptied store shelves of basic items. Food staples, including eggs, rice, beans, and bread were quickly liquidated from store shelves as consumers compulsively purchased multiple items in an effort to stockpile for future use (Islam et al. 2021). Grocery and big box stores were forced to place limits on the number of items consumers purchased in a single visit in order to accommodate the needs of all their customers.

Healthcare providers, government workers, and grocery store employees were deemed essential workers, which allowed their facilities to remain open (Park and Abiad 2020). While some businesses were able to continue to function throughout the pandemic shutdown, others, including restaurants, bars, entertainment venues, gyms, retail stores, banks, malls, libraries, and service providers, such as auto repair shops, closed their doors. Private practice physicians resorted to virtual appointments with their patients, and nonemergency medical procedures were canceled or rescheduled at local hospitals and clinics. Dental offices canceled appointments and closed their doors indefinitely. Government offices were reduced to restrictive access, postponing courthouse business (trials, hearings, etc.) and requiring all visitors to wear a mask upon entering the facilities. With travel placed on hold, post offices that provide passport application services suspended in-person appointments. Vehicle emissions checks, inspections, and property taxes payments were delayed.

With stay-at-home orders in place, fewer individuals occupied highways and roads, resulting in the ideal commute. Unfortunately for the economy, this decrease in traffic impacted businesses and consumer procurement of goods and services (Martin et al. 2020). A decrease in commuting due to the lockdowns negatively affected supply chains in restricting the mobility of workers to transport goods and services to neighboring cities and states (Asahi et al. 2021). Although customer consumption increased during the pandemic with the global lockdowns, product availability became scarce in some areas, causing manufacturers to mass-produce their products for delivery to local stores. This too became a problem due to the travel restrictions; however, companies were able to transport needed goods as a result of identifying as necessary workers and product and service providers.

2.0 Government Intervention and Response

In a study on United States' governors' response to the pandemic, Baccini and Broduer (2021) discovered that politically, states with Democratic governors were more likely to impose a statewide shelter-in-place order than those states with a Republican governor. Likewise, these Democratic governors were quicker to execute these orders, resulting in a more immediate cause and effort on the economy in an effort to place the health and welfare of citizens above the cost of imposing the stay-at-home order. As a result of these extreme measures of shutting down the country, businesses began to suffer great losses in revenue and staff. Government officials closed the borders and restricted travel to and from the United States, which halted the import and export of goods and services and further strained the economy. Attempts were made by organizations to maintain their employees with the supposition that the shutdown would not last long.

The United States government stepped in with the Coronavirus Aid, Relief, and Economic Security Act (CARES) by offering small business loans to companies (Thorbecke 2020). These loans were designed to assist small businesses with continuing to pay their employees, offer tax assistance, and assistance to those who lost their jobs by expanding unemployment benefits. Under the Paycheck Protection Program, individual taxpayers earning less than $75,000 per year and those taxpayers who file jointly making $150,000 or less per year were given funds in an effort to stimulate the economy which was heavily impacted by the pandemic. These stimulus funds were provided for citizens to help with their daily financial responsibilities. Although the funds were a short-term relief to consumers to pay for much-needed expenses, they did very little to break the sting of unemployment or stimulate a badly bruised economy (Thorbecke 2020). In an attempt to further aid the country's need to combat the deadly virus and support essential medical workers, the government increased spending allotted for supplying viral medications, masks, and other personal protection equipment (PPE) needed (Park et al. 2020).

The American Rescue Plan, signed into law on March 11, 2021, by US Pres. Joe Biden was also implemented as additional assistance to citizens affected by the pandemic. The plan included an increase in the Child Tax Credit for those citizens with children as well as assistance with paying rent and making mortgage payments to ensure families would not lose their homes due to an inability to pay when their employment was halted. This plan also provided assistance to small businesses to offset the cost of company payroll taxes and employee tax credits. Individual unemployment compensation was increased as well.

As the rate of infections quickly spread across the United States, the government took further preventative measures to flatten the curve of the daily positive cases, hospitalizations, and deaths due to the pandemic. International flights were canceled, large gatherings were forbidden, schools and institutions of higher education were closed, and visitors were discouraged from entering the country by sealing the borders (Subramaniam and Chakraborty 2021). Likewise, neighboring countries and those beyond the borders of the United States restricted travel from the States into their territories.

2. Job Loss and Unemployment

Businesses providing in-person goods and services encountered the greatest hit in the early days of the pandemic with regard to unemployment rates. Just weeks into the pandemic in April 2020, the US unemployment rate rose to 14.8%, which was one of the highest rates the country had seen since 1948. Industry-wise, perhaps the greatest jolt of the pandemic was felt by the hospitality and leisure industry (Cho and Winters 2020). Limitations on occupancies as well as social distance requirements contributed to these losses as entertainment facilities, sports arenas, restaurants, and bars were closed with no indication of when they might reopen. According to the National Restaurant Association, 3% of restaurants closed their doors for good due to the pandemic between March and June 2020. Approximately $120 billion in revenue was lost in this industry during the first quarter of the pandemic (Song et al. 2021). Likewise, the closing of those businesses deemed nonessential led to an increase in poverty rates as a result of individuals no longer working. A loss of income and a significant decrease in any disposable income these workers may have had resulted in their inability to take care of their families and meet their financial obligations (Li et. al 2021).

With consumers confined to their homes, they could not travel, thus, prompting a severe blow to hotels, restaurants, and vacation resorts. Airports, train stations, and bus depots were shut down, and car rental company parking lots were overrun with rental cars. Summer vacations were on hold, and family get-togethers were canceled. As a result of this reduction in travel, the unemployment rate in the hospitality and leisure industry rose to 39.3%. This increase would not see a decline until eight months after the beginning of the pandemic when it fell to 16.7% in December 2020.

Likewise, the service industry sustained great losses as the need for laundry service and dry cleaning was drastically reduced. Since working remotely afforded employees the flexibility of *dressing down* for work, dry cleaners closed their doors. Personal care facilities, including nail and hair salons and barbershops, closed as local government officials deemed their services as nonessential. These services were put on hold, or consumers were resigned to attend to those needs at home.

With companies implementing remote work options for their employees, construction of new nonresidential buildings and maintenance of existing office space came to a screeching halt as employees vacated their usual work locations. There was no longer a need for daily custodial staff with no employees on the premises, which affected custodial services. Businesses that required employees to work assembly lines were hit hard early in the pandemic with multiple cases of COVID-19 spreading rapidly throughout their plants. Social distancing made it difficult to work in these organizations and subsequently caused employees to vacate their positions.

A significant gap in the unemployment rate statistics was identified when reviewing the educational status of employees. Cho and Winters (2020) discovered that employees holding a bachelor's degree or greater experienced less strain of unemployment than their counterparts who were not educated beyond high school. Those employees with higher education degrees experienced 8.4% of the unemployment rate while high school graduates experienced 21.2% of the unemployment rate. Likewise, full-time employees were less likely to experience unemployment during the pandemic compared to part-time employees. In April 2020, full-time employee unemployment rates were at 12.9% while part-timers' unemployment rates were at 24.5%. Fortunately, with time passing, the gap in unemployment rates between these groups has narrowed.

3. Supply and Demand

One major factor in the direction the economy quickly took shortly after the first couple of weeks of the pandemic is a lack of preparedness. While the general population stockpiled toilet paper, bottled water, cleaning supplies, and Clorox wipes, hospitals and healthcare facilities struggled to obtain necessary PPE for their essential workers (Kaye et al. 2020). PPE, including protective gowns, medical gloves, N95 masks, and respirators were in short supply, and the need for these items grew rapidly each day (Park and Abiad 2020). Hospitals and other healthcare providers shared their resources to protect their essential workers while attending to the influx of COVID-19 patients. Companies whose specialty had little or nothing to do with PPE began mass-producing masks and hand sanitizer, and stores set quantity limits on products in order to maintain on-hand supply.

Consumer panic-buying sent the country in a tailspin, and manufacturers were unable to keep up with the demand for these goods. Essential items were purchased with no regard for an impending consumer shortage (Islam et al. 2021). Consumers stockpiled germ-fighting and disease prevention products, causing an immediate hardship on stores to keep their shelves stocked and manufacturers fell short trying to keep up with the demand. Social media became an important outlet for dispensing news and propaganda regarding where to buy needed products as well as spreading stories of violence against citizens who were able to obtain these products in large quantities. Likewise, social media kept those individuals informed when an impending shortage of goods was inevitable at a given store.

With the country under stay-at-home orders, consumers had to find alternative ways of obtaining the goods and services they traditionally would secure in person. A decrease in the demand for transportation, including city buses and intercity railways, made it possible to give preference to basic and obligatory goods and services (Chien et al. 2021). As one of the most needed essential businesses during a pandemic, grocery stores experienced a surge in online purchases, deliveries, and store pickups. Consumers were now fearful of in-store shopping and began to rely on pickup and delivery services. This change in shopping behaviors led to a 255% increase in pickup services and a 158% increase in delivery services (Chenarides et al. 2020). Like brick-and-mortar grocery stores, online companies, including Amazon, saw a tremendous spike in business with consumers placing online and telephone orders for goods traditionally purchased in stores. Since online and telephone ordering was already in place with some stores, an adjustment in staff was needed to accommodate this increase in online services. This was a small step in easing the pain of the rising unemployment rate.

Amid the shutdowns and closures experienced both in the United States and globally, those organizations that provided electronic entertainment and nondurable household products appeared immune to the pandemic as the demand for these goods and services did not decline; rather, demand increased significantly. Services provided by satellite and cable television providers as well as internet providers saw a substantial increase in demand as workers left their offices and students left schools and returned home to work and learn remotely (Thorbecke 2020). These electronic services, along with nondurable household items (items which are consumed and cannot be reused), were not negatively affected by the pandemic. Examples of nondurable household items include the following:

- cosmetics and personal hygiene products,
- cleaning supplies and laundry detergent,
- beer and spirits,

- cigarettes and tobacco,

- prescription and over-the-counter medication,

- office supplies,

- paper products, including paper towels, toilet paper, and paper plates, and

- plastics, rubber products, and textiles.

As a result of the increased time confined at home, consumer durable goods, including household appliances (refrigerators, washers, and dryers) and electronic devices (televisions, computers, mobile telephones, and tablets), were in high demand during the peak of the pandemic. These items, in connection with electronic entertainment services, became a way of life for consumers globally.

The sharing economy (SE) refers to those services provided to consumers through a system of sharing resources, such as Airbnb, Uber, and Lyft. This sector of the economy produced 6.23 million jobs, and with the onset of COVID-19, the reduction in demand for these services has concerned its service providers, some of which were laid off from their full-time jobs. Pre-pandemic through the SE, consumers used the system to reduce the cost of travel by using the rideshare services of other consumers and renting a room or house for their vacations to save on hotel and resort costs (Hossain 2021). These services are yet another casualty of the pandemic, given the shutdown and suspension of dining out, vacationing, and for many employees, working remotely. The demand for these services drastically decreased among consumers. As a result, many who lost their SE jobs were offered government assistance through stimulus packages. Unfortunately, there was a delay in receiving these funds as many states' procedures were outdated and needed to be updated prior to payout. Meanwhile, those Airbnb service providers who remained active during the pandemic offered essential frontline workers (physicians, nurses, and medical technicians) free room and board to assist in the fight to control the spread of COVID-19.

As a significant factor in the success or failure of the tourism industry, car rental companies suffered substantially. Travel and tourism were brought to a halt as a result of the shelter-in-place orders; however, the need for rental cars remained. Consumers still needed a means of transportation as they put their personal vehicle maintenance on hold due to mechanics and car care facilities shutting their doors and public transportation at a standstill. In response to that need, consumers sought out car rental companies, who, due to the decrease in travel, experienced market volatility. Hertz Car Rentals filed for bankruptcy after a payout to their executives of $16 million in retention bonuses (Nhamo et al. 2020) while employees lost their jobs through layoffs.

The demand for healthcare throughout the pandemic was at an all-time high as communities scrambled to control the spread of the virus. Daily increases in positive COVID-19 cases, hospitalizations, and subsequent deaths put healthcare organizations on high alert as they hastened to make room for the influx of patients needing immediate care. Emergency rooms were inundated with COVID-19 cases and hospital bed capacities were exceeded; however, due to stay-at-home orders, hospitals and clinics experienced fewer traffic accident victims and fatalities (Cavallo and Forman, 2020). This allowed healthcare providers more leeway to attend to their more critical COVID-19 patients.

4. Stock Market Trends

The onset and subsequent prolonged duration of the COVID-19 pandemic affected all aspects of life including the stock market. In the first few months of the pandemic, a connection between the rise in daily positive COVID-19 cases and subsequent deaths was identified (Li et al. 2021). The connection between stock market volatility and the pandemic directly resulted in negative stock returns for investors. Furthermore, in some countries, this connection proved to be a long-range forecast of the extended impact on the stock market returns. This connection continued even after some of the shutdown restrictions were later lifted due to the steady rise of positive cases and deaths. With the global pandemic in full swing, stock markets have displayed diverse degrees of volatility over the past seventeen months (Uddin et al. 2021). Investors were presented with more reason for concern as they watched the markets fluctuate due to economic shutdowns across the globe. Considerable declines in the stock market indexes have contributed to a significant rise in unemployment as nearly 17 million US workers filed for unemployment benefits by early April 2020 (Cavallo, Forman 2020). Researchers have determined that there is a significant negative relationship between the fear of COVID-19 and all that entails and stock market returns during a specific period of time. Since individuals are subject to rely on personal temperaments and feelings when making decisions, including those related to investing, the fear of the pandemic's outcome has disquieted some investors (Subramamiam and Chakraborty 2021). In early 2020, the global economic movement was quickly suspended, and the business sectors most affected were:

- personal services which required face-to-face contact between individuals, including hair salons, barbershops, and nail salons,
- travel and vacations, including cruises, taxis and air transportation, and hotels,
- primary and secondary education, as well as higher education,

- cultural activities, including galleries and sporting events, indoor and outdoor concerts, sports venues, and expos, and
- retail commerce (Buszko et al. 2021).

In other business sectors, cost structures and incomes have changed drastically, and stock futures remain uncertain as there is no clear indication of how much longer the pandemic will last. The steps taken to control the spread of the virus (country and state lockdowns, social distancing, mask mandates, travel restrictions, etc.) have contributed to the fluctuations of the stock market prices. Shifts in trade, healthcare systems, and employment, as well as production, and security policies are predicted to become permanent as a result of the pandemic (Hossain and Rahaman 2021).

Panic spread by the pandemic hit global financial markets hard. Fear of contracting the virus, along with the shock of the rising numbers in positive COVID-19 cases, hospitalizations, and deaths as a result of the virus caused stock prices to fall globally. The British Broadcasting Company (BBC) reported at the end of March 2020 that the Dow Jones Industrial Average declined by 23%, and the Financial Times Stock Exchange (FTSE) declined by 25%, which proved to be the largest quarterly decrease in 34 years. Likewise, Standard and Poor's 500 Index declined by 20%, the greatest decrease in 13 years (Li et al. 2021). The March 2020 stock market crash was one of the greatest historical stock market crashes on record. The gross domestic product (GDP) in the first quarter of 2020 fell to 4.8%, and unemployment climbed to over 20%, both as a result of the historic collapse of the stock market of 26% over a four-day period (Chien et al. 2021). With regard to foreign direct investments (FDI), increases in this economic category generate a positive subsidy to the GDP, resulting in a shortfall of production demand and an increase in the price and propensity to produce more (Li et al. 2021). When compared to the first quarter of 2019, the demand for global worldwide energy by the end of April 2020 saw a 17% decrease. An increase in the concern of the severity of virus cases resulted in significate decreases in stock market daily indexes. The unpredictability of the stock market during these times played an important part in consumer supply and demand, foreign direct investment of goods and services, as well as employee productivity.

A 2020 study about the impact of government involvement on the economy during the pandemic explored how the stock market responded to the following executive initiatives:

- Social distancing—a recommendation of maintaining a distance of six feet or more from individuals who are not members of the same household. In an effort to effectively social distance individuals from others, schools and outdoor venues, restaurants, and entertainment facilities were closed, public transportation was halted, and organizations closed their doors and sent employees home to work remotely.

- Containment and health response—ensuring the public remains current on all data regarding COVID-19 testing, quarantine strategies, and vaccination research. State and local government agencies provided weekly updates on positive cases to the community in the first several months of the pandemic, followed by updates on the vaccination research progress. Subsequently, as vaccines were made available, the public was informed of vaccination locations and encouraged to make an appointment to get their shot.

- Income support packages—subsidies provided to individuals and families to assist with paying rent, monthly mortgages, and utility bills. With some businesses closing as a means of containing the spread of the virus, thousands of employees lost their jobs, creating a need for financial assistance with meeting their basic needs.

The study found that the stock market is both negatively and positively affected by these governmental measures. The expectation of negative connotations of social distancing resulted in adversary results to the stock market. Adversely, the economy indirectly profited from the decrease in the fervency of the COVID-19 outbreaks (Ashraf 2020).

Several industries suffered in the stock market, and most notable was the airline industry. The value of the US dollar invested in the aerospace sector which supplies airplanes for airlines plummeted to 50 cents during the period between February and July 2020 with no immediate rebound over the course of the next several months. Likewise, a dollar invested in the oil sector during the same February to July 2020 period dropped to 45 cents, and production of oil plunged by 30%. In the tourism industry, a dollar invested in casinos or other gambling facilities or organizations saw a plunge in value to 55 cents while the value of the dollar fell to 57 cents in tourism. Fitness centers and consumer lending organizations, including banks, saw a complete shutdown in consumer foot traffic and business, and the dollar invested fell to 58 cents (Thorbecke 2020).

As a result of the governmental and individual responses to the global pandemic and general fear and uncertainty of one's future, product and service demands dramatically decreased and lead to a rise in unemployment. Oil prices decreased due to a drop in consumer need with many employees working remotely, and the entertainment industry was suspended in time. Future stock prices and trading continues on a slow rebound; however, until countries adapt to a new normal that focuses on the health and welfare of their citizens over profits, the rebound will remain stagnant.

5. Survival and Recovery

What will it take for the country and even the world to recover from the effects of this global pandemic? Restoring public faith in healthcare and government officials will take some time after nearly eighteen months of shutdowns and disruptions to normalcy. In a step toward normalcy, countries around the globe have lifted restrictions as positive COVID-19 cases began to increase again. Some US states entered into phased reopening processes to restart the economy as consumer confidence began to increase with vaccinations (Reed et al. 2020). Although some of its citizens are fully vaccinated, there is no clear indication that this will assist in turning the tide on the economy. Fully vaccinated citizens are still sheltering in place for fear of mingling in public with those who still refuse to be vaccinated or wear a mask. It is now up to the policymakers to weigh the importance of public health in contrast to economic trade-offs.

Employees are returning to work as organizations seek to bring back in-person employee collaborations. Likewise, some employers are offering hybrid work schedules to their employees who have proven that they can be productive working remotely. These hybrid work schedules allow for flexibility in working in-person within their assigned work locations and working remotely. This allows for more options for appropriately spacing individuals while they are in the office without the cost of revamping workstations. Consumer buying has been rejuvenated by those who took advantage of the shelter-in-place mandates to save money otherwise spent in an open economy.

6. Conclusion

The pandemic, amid businesses halting and individuals attempting to social distance from others, caused an immense economic shock both in the United States and globally. The continuous duration of the shutdowns produced great economic losses from which businesses continue to struggle to recover. Since states and territories reopened for business, the Center for Disease Control (CDC) is tracking a rise in positive COVID-19 cases across the United States. Mask mandates were lifted as the general population began getting vaccinated, and positive cases, hospitalizations, and daily deaths were on the decline; however, a large portion of the country's citizens remain unvaccinated. Fear and uncertainty of long-range effects of the vaccines continue to plague some unvaccinated citizens who refuse to abide by the CDC guidelines and suggestions. Confusion over whether to still *mask up* in public is a constant battle as some individuals have taken to violence as a way of expressing their individual rights to remain safe or their right to choose to be safe without government intervention. As individuals seek to regain a modicum of normalcy, vaccinations are still readily available to accommodate those who wish to be vaccinated. The CDC contends that the first step to normalcy is for all individuals to become vaccinated; however, with new more contagious strains of the virus spreading rapidly across the United States and the globe, governments are hard-pressed to control the spread beyond its borders. Some states have reinstated mask mandates, making a partial about-face on the pandemic recovery. Contrary to what some may believe, COVID-19 is here to stay. The United States and even the world have yet to recover and rebound from the stranglehold this pandemic has placed on the lives of the world's inhabitants. Regardless of the personal choices made by individuals, and indeed, governmental policies, the consensus should focus on not only personal health risks but also population health risks as we seek to adapt to and function in the new normal post-pandemic.

References

Asahi, K., Undurraga, E. A., Valdés, R., and Wagner, R. 2021. "The effect of COVID-19 on the economy: Evidence from an early adopter of localized lockdowns." *Journal of Global Health*, 11 (January 16). https://doi.org/10.7189/jogh.10.05002

Ashraf, B. N. 2020. "Economic impact of government interventions during the COVID-19 pandemic: International evidence from financial markets." *Journal of Behavioral and Experimental Finance*, 27 (June). https://doi.org/10.1016/j.jbef.2020.100371

Baccini, L., and Brodeur, A. 2020. Explaining governors' response to the COVID-19 pandemic in the United States. *American Politics Research*, 49 (2) (April): 215–220. https://www.iza.org/publications/dp/13137/explaining-governors-response-to-the-COVID-19-pandemic-in-the-united-states

Buszko, M., Orzeszko, W., and Stawarz, M. 2021. "COVID-19 pandemic and stability of stock market—A sectoral approach." *PLOS ONE*, 16 (5) (May 20). https://doi.org/10.1371/journal.pone.0250938

Cavallo, J. J., and Forman, H. P. 2020. The economic impact of the COVID-19 pandemic on radiology practices. *Radiology*, 296 (3) (April 15): 141–144. https://doi.org/10.1148/radiol.2020201495

Chenarides, L., Grebitus, C., Lusk, J. L., and Printezis, I. 2020. Food consumption behavior during the COVID-19 pandemic. *Agribusiness*, 37 (1) (November 27): 44–81. https://doi.org/10.1002/agr.21679

Chien, F., Sadiq, M., Kamran, H. W., Nawaz, M. A., Hussain, M. S., and Raza, M. 2021. "Co-movement of energy prices and stock market return: environmental wavelet nexus of COVID-19 pandemic from the USA, Europe, and China." *Environmental Science and Pollution Research*, 1–15. https://doi.org/10.1007/s11356-021-12938-2

Cho, S. J., and Winters, J. V. 2020. *The Distributional Impacts of Early Employment Losses from COVID-19* (Discussion paper) (May). IZA Institute of Labor Economics. https://dx.doi.org/10.2139/ssrn.3608515

Hossain, M. 2021. "The effect of the COVID-19 on sharing economy activities." *Journal of Cleaner Production, 280* (1). https://doi.org/10.1016/j.jclepro.2020.124782

Hossain, S., and Rahaman, M. 2021 (February). "The post COVID-19 global economy: An econometric analysis." *IOSR Journal of Economics and Finance,* 12 (1): 22–43. https://www.iosrjournals.org/iosr-jef/papers/Vol12-Issue1/Ser-6/D1201062243.pdf

Islam, T., Pitafi, A. H., Arya, V., Wang, Y., Akhtar, N., Mubarik, S., and Xiaobei, L. 2021. "Panic buying in the COVID-19 pandemic: A multi-country examination." *Journal of Retailing and Consumer Services,* 59 (March). https://doi.org/10.1016/j.jretconser.2020.102357

Kaye, A. D., Okeagu, C. N., Pham, A. D., Silva, R. A., Hurley, J. J., Arron, B. L., Sarfraz, N., Lee, H. N., Ghali, G. E., Gamble, J. W., Liu, H., Urman, R. D., and Cornett, E. M. 2020. "Economic Impact of COVID-19 Pandemic on Health Care Facilities and Systems: International Perspectives." *Best Practice and Research Clinical Anaesthesiology,* 35 (3) (October): 293–306. https://doi.org/10.1016/j.bpa.2020.11.009

Li, W., Chien, F., Kamran, H. W., Aldeehani, T. M., Sadiq, M., Nguyen, V. C., and Taghizadeh-Hesary, F. 2021. "The nexus between COVID-19 fear and stock market volatility." *Economic Research-Ekonomska Istraživanja*, 1–22. https://doi.org/10.1080/1331677X.2021.1914125

Martin, A., Markhvida, M., Hallegatte, S., and Walsh, B. 2020. "Socioeconomic impacts of COVID-19 on household consumption and poverty." *Economics of disasters and climate change, 4* (3) (July 23): 453–479. https://doi.org/10.1007/s41885-020-00070-3

Park, C. Y., Villafuerte, J., Abiad, A., Narayanan, B., Banzon, E., Samson, J. N. G., Aftab, A., and Tayag, M. C. 2020. *An Updated Assessment of the Economic Impact of COVID-19* (May). Asian Development Bank. https://doi.org/10.22617/BRF200144-2

Reed, S., Gonzalez, J. M., and Johnson, F. R. 2020. Willingness to accept trade-offs among COVID-19 cases, social-distancing restrictions, and economic impact: A nationwide US study. *Value in Health,* 23 (11) (November 23): 1438–1443. https://dx.doi.org/10.1016%2Fj.jval.2020.07.003

Song, H. J., Yeon, J., and Lee, S. 2021. Impact of the COVID-19 pandemic: Evidence from the US restaurant industry. *International Journal of Hospitality Management,* 92 (January). https://doi.org/10.1016/j.ijhm.2020.102702

Subramaniam, S., and Chakraborty, M. 2021. "COVID-19 fear index: does it matter for stock market returns?" *Review of Behavioral Finance,* 13 (1): 40–50. https://doi.org/10.1108/RBF-08-2020-0215

Thorbecke, W. 2020. "The impact of the COVID-19 pandemic on the US Economy: Evidence from the stock market." *Journal of Risk and Financial Management,* 13 (10): 233. https://doi.org/10.3390/jrfm13100233

Uddin, M., Chowdhury, A., Anderson, K., and Chaúdhuri, K. 2021. "The effect of COVID–19 pandemic on global stock market volatility: Can economic strength help to manage the uncertainty?" *Journal of Business Research,* 128, 31–44. https://doi.org/10.1016/j.jbusres.2021.01.061

Walmsley, T., Rose, A., and Wei, D. 2021. "The Impacts of the Coronavirus on the economy of the United States." *Economics of Disasters and Climate Change,* 5 (1): 1–52. https://doi.org/10.1007/s41885-020-00080-1

World Health Organization. 2021. *Listings of WHO's Response to* COVID-19 (January 29). https://www.who.int/news/item/29-06-2020-covidtimeline

CHAPTER 5

Impact of COVID-19 on Technology Startups and Technology Entrepreneurship in India

by Deepal Joshi

Abstract

Exogenous shocks disturb business practices and processes. COVID-19, as a global pandemic, is one such shock. Covid-19 marks the beginning of an era of disruptive, continuous and rapid changes in every sector – globally and in India too. India is the third largest technology entrepreneurship ecosystem in the world. Amidst this backdrop, this study discusses the impact of COVID-19 on technology start-ups and technology entrepreneurship in India. The immediate impact of this global pandemic on technology entrepreneurship includes a discussion on the high growth sectors in India during COVID-19, the funding scenario, innovative solutions and philanthropy activities carried on by technology start-ups to combat the pandemic, the challenges faced and survival strategies designed by technology start-ups and the Government of India support to technology start-ups during the pandemic. The long-term impact of this global pandemic on technology entrepreneurship entails a discussion on how COVID-19 accelerated mass digitalization in India, future impact on select technologies in India, sustainability strategies for technology entrepreneurship and the role of resilience and favorable ecosystem in building and sustaining technology entrepreneurship in India. A collection of global research on how technology startups and technology entrepreneurship is likely to be impacted by COVID-19 is presented. This study provides several significant insights for the future of technology entrepreneurship in India, given the changes COVID-19 brought to it.

Keywords: COVID-19, Technology Entrepreneurship, Startups, India, Growth, Sustainability, Policy Measures

INTRODUCTION

1.1 COVID-19: A Global Crisis

On March 11, 2020, the World Health Organisation (WHO) declared the coronavirus generated condition COVID-19 as a global pandemic (WHO, 2020). This led to a phase of uncertainty followed by an explosion of futuristic thinking about what would it mean for the governments, healthcare operations, businesses, education and the humankind at large. All of them have tried to develop alternatives to mitigate damages, prepare, intervene, recover, and rebuild their systems due to the onset and spread of this global pandemic crisis.

Crises like wars, terrorism acts, civil unrest, natural disasters, economic downturns and pandemics are exogenous shocks that disturb the routine business practices and processes. COVID-19 is one such black swan event in the history of humankind. "It is at once an accelerant, an irritant, and a stress test. Its effects will ebb and flow and hit various nations and populations in different ways and on differing timescales. It is this unevenness and unpredictability that defines the challenges ahead." (Brannen, Ahmed & Newton, 2020). The basic assessment of this crisis situation is that COVID-19 is highly disruptive in the short-term, and highly unpredictable in the medium to long-term future.

1.2 How Covid-19 is likely to shape Changes in Technology & Information Technology Sector?

This global pandemic marks the beginning of an era of disruptive, continuous and rapid changes in every sector. Brannen, Ahmed & Newton (2020) discuss how COVID-19 will reshape the future for population, resources, technology, information technology, economics, security and governance. Table 1 depicts what is likely to evolve on the technology and information technology fronts in terms of immediate and long-term effects; triggered by COVID-19.

Table 1. Immediate and Long-term Impacts of COVID-19 on Technology and Information Technology Sectors

Sector	Indicator	Immediate Impacts	Long-term Impacts
Technology	Robotics	Increased interest in robotics due to shortage of public health and labour services	Increased replacement of human labour across sectors (e.g. health, education, food etc.)
	Additive Manufacturing	Rapid production of medical components at points of need	Replacement of standard manufacturing processes with additive technologies (e.g. for health care equipment)
	Internet of Things (IoT)	IoT usage persists high with specific sectors having higher data inflows	Increased dependence on IoT in daily life, especially for health monitoring and surveillance
	Artificial Intelligence (AI)	Rapid adoption of AI chatbots and other AI services to fill sudden requirements	Higher Research & Development (R&D) budgets related to AI and digitalization pushes up adoption across sectors
	Biotechnology	Escalated investment in synthetic biology in seeking therapeutics and vaccines	Growing world-wide competition for leadership in biotechnology; higher national investment in biotech
Information Technology	Access/Privacy	Wide-scale use of digital surveillance to track COVID-19	Increased digital surveillance by nations and businesses
	Data Growth	Wide-scale digitalization of business and social activities	Rapid growth in data volume, emphasis on being or going 'online'
	False News & Social Media	'Infodemic' races ahead of pandemic	Higher geopolitical rivalry in misinformation/ disinformation
	Knowledge & Learning	Large scale adoption of online learning	The digital divide between nations and societies increases inequality

Source: Brannen, Ahmed & Newton, 2020

Given the massive immediate and long-term impacts that this global pandemic is likely to have on the technology and information technology, it will have a significant and direct impact on technology entrepreneurship.

1.3 COVID-19 Crisis, Technology Entrepreneurship and India

Entrepreneurship is an act of being an entrepreneur, or "the owner or manager of a business enterprise who, by risk and initiative, attempts to make profits" (Hisrich, Peters & Shepherd, 2017; Venkataraman & Shane, 2000). Startup founder(s) are generally termed as entrepreneurs for their capacity of designing, launching and running a new business. Crises and entrepreneurship are inter-linked. The effects of COVID-19 pandemic, as a global crisis, are largely negative in nature and devastating in several cases. Entrepreneurship research and entrepreneurship practice address these effects in terms of failure, resilience and crisis management (Amankwah-Amoah, Khan & Wood, 2021; Portuguez Castro & Gomez Germeno, 2020; Kuckertz, Brandle, Gaudig, Hinderer, Reyes, Prochotta et al., 2020). Contrasting with this line of discussion, this study focuses on how COVID-19 is an enabler and growth- promoter of entrepreneurship, technology entrepreneurship specifically.

High-tech entrepreneurship or technological entrepreneurship is defined as the setting up of new enterprises by individuals or corporations to exploit technological innovation (Gupta, Jain, Kusre & Momaya, 2015). Technology entrepreneurship differs from general entrepreneurship to the extent that it focuses on technology-based opportunities that require thorough technological as well as managerial capabilities (Tripathi & Brahma, 2017). Technology entrepreneurship has contributed to a high degree of innovation, job creation and economic development in the developed economies, especially the USA. Apart from US, Canada in North America; UK, Germany, France, Turkey etc. in Europe; Israel, China, India, Japan, Singapore, South Korea etc. among Asian economies and the Australian sub-continent has experienced the emergence and growth of technology entrepreneurship. In 2019, more than 50% of start-ups across the globe were technology based - Web services and apps (18.6%), Software as a service (15.3%), E-commerce (10.1%) and IT and Software (8.6%) (Source: https://valuer.ai/blog/top-50-best-startup-cities/, 2019).

For India, there is a strong realisation that it needs to leverage on its innovative potential through change-driven fast and all-inclusive growth, if it wants to achieve social and economic transformation (Joshi & Achuthan, 2018). Technology entrepreneurship and high-tech start-ups can be the key to achieving this transformation for India. India is the third largest technology entrepreneurial ecosystem in the world. In 2019, the total number of new high-tech start-ups was around 1,300 taking the total number of high-tech start-ups in India to over 9,000. Eight unicorns were added to the Indian high-tech start up ecosystem in 2019. These start-ups created an estimated 60,000 direct and 1.3-1.8 lakh indirect jobs (Joshi, 2021). However, funding and scalability continue to be the major challenges to overcome for technology start-ups in India and globally as well (Bala Subrahmanya, 2015).

The Indian technology entrepreneurship picture looks quite encouraging in the midst of COVID-19 crisis. In 2020, India added more than 1,600 technology start-ups taking the total number to over 12,500. 24 new unicorns were added to the list for India from the period ranging from April 2020 to June 2021. Technology entrepreneurship attracted new investments, created new employment avenues, generated revenue and growth for India during a situation of pandemic.

Amidst this backdrop, this study discusses how technology entrepreneurship is evolving in India through the opportunities provided and challenges posed by the COVID-19 crisis. This chapter is further divided into following sections. The second section discusses the immediate impacts of COVID-19 on technology entrepreneurship in the Indian context. It includes

- The High Growth Sectors in Technology Startups in India amidst COVID-19
- Funding for Technology Entrepreneurship during pandemic situation in India
- Innovative Solutions and Philanthropy Activities by Technology Startups
- Challenges Faced and Survival Strategies designed by Technology Startups
- Government Policy Measures Support for Technology Start-ups during COVID-19 in India

The third section highlights the long-term impacts of this pandemic on technology entrepreneurship in India. It includes

- 'New Normal' and Large-Scale Digitalization in India
- Long-term Consequences of COVID-19 in Specific Technology Sectors
- Sustainability Strategies for Technology Entrepreneurship in India
- Resilience and Favourable Ecosystem - the key elements to Building and Sustaining Technology Entrepreneurship

The fourth section presents a snapshot of global research on how technology startups are likely to be impacted by COVID-19. The chapter concludes with a discussion on significant insights from the study.

2. IMMEDIATE IMPACT OF COVID-19 ON TECHNOLOGY STARTUPS AND TECHNOLOGY ENTREPRENEURSHIP IN INDIA

A pandemic situation like this one is highly disruptive in the short-term and hence this section of the chapter tries to throw light on its immediate impact on the technology startups and technology entrepreneurship in the Indian context. The discussion in this section encompasses the booming technology startup sectors in India during the pandemic, the funding scenario for technology startups, the innovative solutions provided by technology entrepreneurship to combat COVID-19 in India, the short-term challenges faced by technology startups and government support to technology entrepreneurship during COVID-19.

1.1 High Growth Sectors in Technology Startups in India amidst COVID-19

Year 2020 and 2021 witnessed a significant rise in the number of technology startups and a phenomenal growth in the existing technology startups in several sectors. COVID-19 has proved to be an external enabler of technology entrepreneurship in this context. The rise of technology entrepreneurship in these sectors is touching future expectations. Figures 1, 2, 3, 4, 5 and 6 explain the reasons for growth and some significant developments during 2020 and 2021 in fintech, edtech, healthtech, online retail, Software as a Service (SaaS) and remote working tools, Over-The-Top (OTT) platforms, online gaming and vernacular podcasting respectively in India amidst the COVID-19 crisis. This discussion is a part of immediate impact as we are able to gauge the effects of only 15 months on these technology startup sectors – From March 2020 to June 2021.

Figure 1. Fintech Entrepreneurship in India during COVID-19	
Reasons for growth of Fintech	**Notable developments during 2020 and 2021**
• Convenience of technlogy use and fear of infection from handling cash are two major reasons attributing to the growth of fintech • Digital payments was a nice idea pre - COVID; it has shifted to being an essential service; consumers prefer digital payments for groceries, utility etc. • Within fintech, apart from payment, wealth management, insurance, credit scoring, and regtech are growth drivers	• India attracted $2.7 billion investment in fintech in 2020; second highest after $3.5 billion in 2019 • Upto 2020, one-third unicorns in the technology startup space were from fintech - Paytm being the highest valued fintech startup • Digital payment app PhonePe captured a little over 40 percent market share of the UPI market as the number one player for January 2021 • Newer opportunities within fintech include inter-operability enablers, alternative investment assets, revenue flow-based financing, and SaaS financing
Source: Prepared by author based on Rao, Goyal, Kumar, Hassan & Shahimi, 2021; PTI, 2021	

Figure 2. Edtech Entrepreneurship in India during COVID-19	
Reasons for growth of Edtech	**Notable developments during 2020 and 2021**
•People skeptical to send their children to schools/colleges where social distancing cannot be practiced •Edtech topped not only user growth and Venture Capital (VC) funding but Twitter trends and Google searches too, in 2020 •Edtech startups recorded robust growth in traffic, engagement, subscriptions and renewals in contrast to previous struggles to attrach users. The scepticism around e-learning declined, and it went mainstream •Growth sectors in edtech include Video/live and gamified learning, virtual class tools, tutor/institute discovery, student performance analytics, and corporate L&D while emerging opportunities include immersive learning solutions, vocational courses, smart education campuses, and outcome-linked coaching solutions	•Edtech startups raised a total of $2.2 billion,in 2020 as compared to $522 million in 2019; meaning a 4.2X growth •K-12 and test preparation startups received the largest share of edtech startup funding in India during this period • BYJU'S ,India's highest valued edtech unicorn, had 45 million free users on the platform with 3.5 million paid subscribers within a period of 2015 to March 2020 –By the end of 2020, the number went up to 70 million users and 4.7 million subscribers •Unicorn edtech startups such as Byju's and Unacademy, other notable edtech startups such as Vedantu, Convegenius, Toppr, Precisely etc. and 2020-born edtech startups such as Learnvern, Skillovilla, BeyondSkool, Filo received funding and witnessed growth

Source: Prepared by author based on Godha & Sharma, 2021.

Mitter, 2021; Singh, Adebayo, Saini & Singh, 2021

Figure 3. Healthtech Entrepreneurship in India during COVID-19

Reasons for growth of Healthtech	Notable developments during 2020 and 2021
• Reduction in physical or in-person OPD by senior or aged doctors and transition to tele-consultations • Tele-consultation is more sought after by patients to avoid risk of infections and over-crowded hospitals • Novel guidelines for telemedicine practice issued by the Government of India in March 2020 to facilitate medical advice for chronic patients who have routine healthcare needs • Notification by The Insurance Regulatory and Development Authority (IRDA) advising the insurers to allow telemedicine coverage under health insurance programmes • COVID-19 has altered the view of technology for both healthcare providers and consumers. Additional emerging use cases include digital tools for small/medium sized care providers, neurology and neurosciences, low cost connected devices for screening, and emergency care	• From being online pharmacies, health tech startups moved to providing Voice Artificial Intelligence (AI) feature, Telemedicine, e-consultation, e-prescription and electronic medical records • 2.2X growth in telemedicine/teleconsultation platforms, a 1.8X increase in usage of electronic health record systems, and a 2.5X growth in active households witnessed by online pharmacy startups during 2020 • Healthtech sector recorded 77 deals raising \$455 Mn in funding in 2020 against \$512 Mn funding in 62 deals in 2019. This trend should continue in 2021, with more news of new funding and announcements of mergers & acquisitions • The telemedicine market in India is expected to grow at a Compounded Annual Growth Rate (CAGR) of 31 per cent for the period 2020-25 and reach \$5.5 billion • Reliance acquired 60% stake in Netmeds and 100% stake in its subsidiaries, healthtech startups like Curefit, 1mg, IVF access, Healthpix, Phable etc. raised fresh funding in 2020 • Online pharmacy unicorn Pharmeasy acquired Medlife in May 2021 to become India's largest e-pharma company

Source: Prepared by author based on Dash, 2020; Anupam, 2021. Narayanan, 2021

Figure 4. Online Retail Entrepreneurship in India during COVID-19

Reasons for growth of Online Retail	Notable developments during 2020 and 2021
• Offline retail was badly hit during COVID-19 paving way for more online retail especially in groceries • New opportunities in omnichannel formats, social commerce, warehousing innovations, faster delivery etc. continue to emerge	• Online retail giants such as Flipkart and Amazon, growing players like JioMart, BigBasket, Grofers etc. witnessed increase in app downloads and user volumes • Online retailers in fashion, ethnic wear, formal footwear etc. categories experienced phases of reduced sales during COVID-19

Source: Prepared by author based on Kaur & Sahdev, 2020.

Rakshit, Islam, Mondal & Paul, 2021

Figure 5. SaaS and Remote-Working Tools Entrepreneurship in India during COVID-19

Reasons for growth of SaaS and Remote-working Tools	Notable developments during 2020 and 2021
• Work From Home (WFH) emerged as the buzz word during COVID-19 generating high requirement for SaaS and remote-working tools • SaaS and remote-working tools facilitate the ongoing projects and pave the road map for future endeavours to greater extent • Businesses have announced their support for partial remote work policy even after COVID-19 subsides • Startups offer software to support functions such as payroll processing, computer-aided design, accounting, customer relationship management (CRM), management information systems (MIS), invoicing, human resource management, talent acquisition, content management, geographic information systems (GIS) etc.	• Remote functions require SaaS tools and the Indian SaaS market is slated to grow to over $20 billion in 2022 from around $6 billion in 2019 • 20 percent of VC and Private Equity (PE) funding in the Indian tech startup ecosystem in India during 2020 went to SaaS startups • Examples of SaaS based startups witnessing growth in 2020 include Flock, an office team communication software firm; Facilion, a Chennai based IoT SaaS startup for property management; Snapbizz, a firm providing billing software for Goods & Services Tax (GST) • Business giants such as Jio Platforms, Microsoft and Facebook launched remote-working tools

Source: Prepared by author based on Bhattacharya, 2020

Figure 6. OTT Platforms, Online Gaming and Vernacular Podcasting Entrepreneurship in India during COVID-19

Reasons for growth of OTT Platforms, Online Gaming & Vernacular Podcasting	Notable Developments in 2020 and 2021
•Time and cost efficient enterntainment for homebound individuals with few leisure activities to participate in •Personalized entertainment experience from the comfort of homes • User engagement in online gaming escalated, gaming activity throughout the day with peak between 8 pm to midnight witnessed •India is a country with 22 modern Indian languages, 720 recognized dialects • Increased demand for information in vernacular languages	•60% growth in OTT subscription in India during COVID-19. Time spent per day and subscription amount spent per month on OTT platforms increased 2X • While Netflix and Amazon Prime were already popular, Indian OTT platforms such as Voot, Hotstar, Zee5, AltBalaji, JioCinema gained traction • Indian gaming companies such as WinZo Games & Paytm First Games experienced increased user base, more customer engagement etc. •33 percent growth rate in vernacular podcasting in 2020 • Example is growth of Khabri, a vernacular online platform, for content from news, to mythological series, fun stories, and poems, and even educational

Source: Prepared by author based on Amin, Griffiths & Dsouza, 2020. Madnani, Fernandes & Madnani, 2020; Sheth, 2020

1.1 Funding for Technology Startups during COVID-19 in India

Based on literature review and expert opinions from various start-ups in India, Sreenivasan and Suresh (2021) identify eight enablers for start-ups in India. This study indicates 'sufficient funds' as the most critical enabler. The access to financing sources is critical for start, survival and sustainability of start-ups, including the technology start-ups – globally and in the Indian context, also. Financing for startups becomes a significant issue during COVID-19. "This pandemic adds a destructive effect to the financing issue, impacting banks, investors and public institutions across countries." Villaseca, Navio-Marco and Gimeno, 2020, pg. 2. Therefore, financing is a crucial factor as an immediate impact of this pandemic on technology start-ups and technology entrepreneurship in India. In this context, the author tries to discuss the scenario of financing from March 2020 to June 2021 for technology start-ups during the COVID-19 pandemic in India.

Fresh investments amounting to $9.33 billion were reported in the technology start up sector in India up to December 2020. Figure 7 provides a comparative scenario of total funding generated and the number of funding rounds in technology start-ups in India during a five-year period from 2016 to 2020. It can be observed that although the number of funding rounds fell to its lowest in five years in 2020, the amount raised was higher than 2016 and 2017 -- when investors chipped in $3.51 billion and $6.43 billion, respectively. This signals continued investor interest in technology start-ups during 2020 (Shah, 2020).

Figure 7. Five Years Comparative Picture of Total Funding in Billion Dollars and Number of Funding Rounds for Technology Start-ups in India

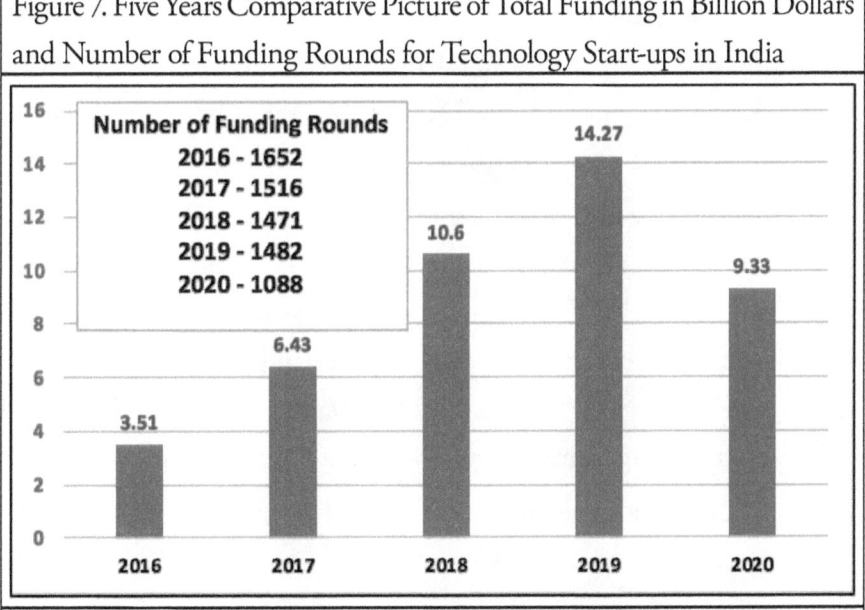

Source: Prepared by author based on Shah (2020)

Some salient features of funding for technology start-ups in India during a period of March 2020 to June 2021 (NASSCOM (The National Association of Software and Service Companies), 2020; Shah, 2020) are discussed below:

- Year 2020 was divided into two distinct halves for Venture Capital Financiers (VCFs) – the first six months witnessed significant reduction in fresh funding though portfolio companies were supported by VCFs. The other six months of 2020 saw businesses returning to the 'new normal' with ongoing pandemic situation and technology entrepreneurship attempted exploiting new opportunities with increased funding activity towards the end of 2020.

- Most noteworthy VCFs who have funded technology start-ups in India during this period are Accel, Falcon Edge, Lets Venture, Lightspeed Venture Partners, Matrix Partners, Steadview Capital, Sequoia Capital and Tiger Global.

- Technology entrepreneurship in India received a shot in the arm; fuelled by new opportunities generated by COVID-19. Significant venture capital investments on seed and Series A deals were reported. Seed stage investment deals grew by 50% in 2020; as compared to 2019.

- Technology start-ups in sectors like Fast Moving Consumer Goods (FMCGs) and fashion e-commerce, automobiles and travel tech struggled with zero cashflow, while areas such as edtech, grocery e-commerce, hyperlocal delivery, SaaS and remote working tools and healthtech flourished, experiencing a never-before surge in traction, engagement as well as investor confidence.

- There were differences in the funding pattern of technology start-ups between 2019 and 2020. During 2019, there were 28 rounds of over $100 million funding, which reduced to

24 rounds in 2020. However, these rounds generated $4.71 billion worth of funding. Large funding deals were seen for start-ups such as Byju's, Unacademy, Zomato, Cred, Delhivery, Razorpay, PhonePe, Ecom Express, Vedantu and Cars24.

- The geographical distribution of the funding during 2020 followed the trend of previous years. Bengaluru, Delhi NCR and Mumbai accounted for more than 90 percent of the start-up investments in the country, reiterating the high concentration of favourable elements for technology entrepreneurship ecosystem in these cities. Bengaluru led with $4.3 billion in start-up investments (Start-up Genome, 2020), followed by Delhi NCR ($3 billion) and Mumbai ($2 billion).

- Several corporates and strategic investors went for mergers and acquisitions in the technology start up sector in India during 2020 and 2021. The acquisition of WhiteHat Jr. for $300 million by Byju's; the acquisition of online furniture retailer Urban Ladder for $24 million and online pharmacy Netmeds for $83 million by Reliance Industries Limited, acquisition of Medlife by Pharmeasy for an estimated $240 million are significant.

1.1 Technology Entrepreneurship provides Innovative Solutions and Philanthropy Activities to tackle COVID-19

One of the most significant immediate impacts of this pandemic situation in India has been the way in which technology entrepreneurs and investors honed their problem-solving skills and helped develop solutions to tackle COVID-19 and assist the front line workers in combating the situation. Technology startups teamed up to make several technology-driven ideas into feasible solutions. Some significant developments from technology entrepreneurship for providing innovative solutions to tackle COVID-19 in India are discussed in Table 2.

Table 2. Innovative Solutions by Technology Start-ups to Combat COVID-19 in India

Category	Specific Solutions	Examples of Tech Start-ups From India
COVID-19 Surveillance Tools	Smart cameras, drones, goggles etc. to ensure social distancing	Contatrack, Cyran AI Solutions
	Crowd management, movement detection, geofencing to check if required protocols were followed at public places and to enforce quarantine protocols for suspected and confirmed COVID-19 patients	Heamac, TechGropse, Technodom
	Drones for surveillance, sanitization, delivery etc.	Garuda Aerospace, Redwing
COVID-19 Prevention Tools	Disinfection Services	Scitech Airon, My Ventures
	Technology based large scale production of Personal Protective Equipment (PPE) kits, masks	Sahas, E-spin Nanotech
COVID-19 Supportive Service Tools	Simple delivery solutions to enable safe and prompt delivery	Meru, Ola, Rapido
	Hotels converted to quarantine centres	Oyo
COVID-19 Testing and Health Monitoring Tools	COVID-19 testing kits and centres	E-spin Nanotech, 1mg, Healthians, Klinicapp
	Tech-based health monitoring systems	Portea, Zealth, CogniCare
	Ventilators and other respiratory support	InnAccel, Nocca Robotics
Mental Health Counselling Tools during COVID-19	Solutions for mental wellness	Innerhour, Your Dost, ePsyclinic
	COVID-19 helplines	Haqdarshak, StepOne, COVID-19 response

Source: Prepared by author based on Bhalla (2020)

This situation triggered a wave of acts of generosity and philanthropy by technology start-ups in India. Technology entrepreneurs and investors from India provided prompt response to fight COVID-19 by creating several funds. These funds:

- Work with the government and other significant stakeholders to escalate the development of innovative ideas which can tackle the pandemic outbreak (e.g. Action COVID-19 Team – ACT)

- Work towards mental wellness counselling for technology start-up founders and employees (e.g. COVID-19 SaasBOOMi Fund)

- Provide financial support for start-ups working to combat COVID-19 (e.g. AngelList's COVID-19 Relief Fund)

- Organise online hackathon for start-ups to promote development of COVID-19 solutions (e.g. Wingify's hackathon)

One immediate impact of COVID-19 is the response of technology giants to provide the much-needed help to Indians on specific fronts in the fight against the pandemic (Mittal & Shah, 2021). The succeeding discussion provides several such examples:

- Fintech unicorn Paytm - raised funds internally for procuring 10,000 oxygen concentrators. Later, it opened the fundraiser to its users and matched donations of those who contribute to procure 20 to 30 thousand oxygen concentrators during the second COVID-19 wave in India.

- Logistics and supply chain unicorn Delhivery - provided logistical support on a subsidised basis for importing oxygen concentrators from China at a time when India had been hit by a shortage of air cargo capacity.

- Food delivery unicorn Zomato - Zomato's non-profit arm Zomato Feeding India collaborated with Delhivery to raise Rs. 50 crores for medical supplies.

- Online pharmacy unicorn Pharmeasy - Used its network of 80,000 retailers and 5,000 distributors across the country to accelerate the drive for vaccination against COVID-19.

- Online travel company EaseMyTrip - Imported oxygen concentrators to rent and to distribute free of cost to hospitals.

- Payment gateway Razorpay - Helped not-for-profit organisations collect donations for assisting Covid-19 patients by activating their payments page within 24 hours and not charging transaction fee on donations up to Rs. 10 lakhs.

- Sheroes, a women-only social network, with ACT Grants & Project StepOne - Created a pool of volunteers to help bridge the gap between the doctors and patients by offering and verifying information and supporting calls.

- Vivekananda Hallekere, cofounder of the dockless two-wheeler rental solution start up Bounce and Venture Capitalist Prakhar Khanduja – Created a public group on WhatsApp named 'Donation - India', for sharing requests by people who faced shortages to afford treatment for Covid-19; accepting donations as small as Rs. 100.

- Ashish Singhal, cofounder of crypto investment platform Coinswitch -pledged $1 million Action COVID-19 Team (ACT) grants; Pravin Jadhav, founder of Raise Financial Services, pledged $50,000.

- Sandeep Nailwal, cofounder of blockchain scalability platform Polygon -started accepting payments in cryptocurrency Ethereum and raised $1 million plus for fighting COVID-19 in India.

2.4 Challenges Faced and Survival Strategies Adopted by Technology Start-ups in India during COVID-19

Due to their small size start-ups have limited resources, making then more vulnerable to the internal and external shocks such as: financial issues, losing a critical employee, entry to new market, financial crisis or a pandemic (Eggers, 2020; Simo'n-Moya, Revuelto-Taboada & Ribeiro-Soriano, 2016). COVID-19 was certainly an external shock for technology start-ups and technology entrepreneurship in India. It created several challenges for start-ups in the short-term (Amankwah-Amoah, Khan & Wood, 2021). However, technology start-ups designed survival strategies to overcome each of these challenges. Table 3 and 4 provide a snapshot of the challenges faced and survival strategies designed by technology start-ups in India to sustain during this global pandemic situation.

The first column of tables 3 and 4 shows the challenge faced by the technology start-ups during COVID-19 in India. The second column provides the details of the challenge and the third column describes the survival strategies devised by technology start-ups and technology entrepreneurs. These challenges are not exclusive to, but definitely applicable to technology entrepreneurship in India in the COVID-19 context.

Table 3. Challenges and Survival Strategies of Technology Startups during COVID-19 in India – Part 1

Challenge	Details of the Challenge	Survival Strategies Adopted
Technology	• Transition in work style due to COVID-19 such as mandatory Work From Home (WFH) • Employees moved to their hometowns during long phases of lockdown leading to internet connectivity issues • Lack of physical access to critical infrastructure such as workshops or labs	• Tech startups practised voluntary WFH even before COVID-19; which made transition easier for them compared to others • Pre-existing high levels of technology expertise and adoption helped • Startups operating on cloud computing did not face issues of access to critical infrastructure and others adapted to collaborative technologies
Finance	• Clients delayed payments and sought liberal payment terms • During the initial phase of COVID-19 induced lockdown, there were apprehensions about startup funding and 65% of technology startups faced a significant impact on funding • VC exits declined by about 70% to $1.3 billion in 2020 from $4.4 billion in 2019 due to the adverse effect of pandemic and the VC portfolios not reaching maturity	• Startups tried to adapt to prioritizing relations with clients and foregoing current revenues to some extent in anticipation of better business prospects in future • Most of the tech startups faced major funding crisis from March to June 2020. This was followed by a period of steady rise in interest of venture capitalists and angel investors for funding. COVID-19 triggered situations where most of the tech startups experienced a promising growth

Supply Chain Disruptions	• Startups dealing with tangible products such as B2C e-commerce faced supply chain disruptions. Lockdown and fear of people about contracting COVID-19 led to this situation • Restrictions of inter-state and inter-country mobility further deepened the supply chain crisis. Advance payment received from clients had to be returned due to inability to deliver • Startups operating in non-essential goods categories were the worst hit due to lack of demand	• Startups tried to tap alternate sources of supply to plan deliveries for clients. Technology based startups in the field of logistics designed solutions for safe and prompt delivery • Tech startups focused on high adoption of some specific products and services in the short run to overcome the temporary situation

Source: Adapted from Eggers 2020 and Jha 2020

Table 4. Challenges and Survival Strategies of Technology Startups during COVID-19 in India – Part 2

Challenge	Details of the Challenge	Survival Strategies Adopted
Communication	• Virtual connection to clients and intermediaries created barriers for startup entrepreneurs and leaders to judge people and make decisions. There was lack of aid to observation of attitude, body language, expressions and the physical setup of the client/intermediary's workplace. Closing of deals reduced inspite of continued negotiations • Indian culture lays emphasis on exchanging gifts and expressing positive emotions to close deals and build relationships. This became difficult due to COVID-19	• Startups provided discounts to their clients/intermediaries who were facing tough financial conditions • This meant a strategy of prioritizing personal relationships with clients in order to improve future business prospects, even foregoing short-term gains
Issues with New Recruits	• Contrary to the global situation of massive layoffs and high unemployment rates due to COVID-19, technology startups engaged in hiring employees to meet new demands and growth. These new employees underwent virtual induction into the organisations; with no physical meetings with their teams • This created issues of judging capabilities of new employees and difficulty in providing the guidance they need during the initial periods	• Startup entrepreneurs and HR departments ensured that new recruits had the hardware, software and office supplies as required. They were providing thorough training on using virtual work tools

		• New hires were explained the departmental culture through several virtual meetings and their supervisors were asked to set specific goals and expectations for new recruits to judge their capabilities • Frequent virtual meetings and mentoring sessions were arranged
Employee Engagement and Retention	• Entrepreneurs/Leaders find it difficult to manage and motivate teams. Technology startups required odd hours of working and the homes of employees were not ready for such office environment. Data theft was also a probable risk • Startups have lesser defined procedures and routines as compared to established businesses and it became more challenging during COVID-19 times	• Founders/leaders played a significant role in employee engagement and check-in with employees • Leaders in the startup team had to spend more time in clarifying temporary roles for their teams • There were startups using (e.g.) 'decentralised gamified work environments' to positively motivate the employees doing better and even demote employees not working up to the mark

Source: Adapted from Eggers 2020 and Jha 2020

1.5 Government Policy Measures Support for Technology Start-ups during COVID-19 in India

The onset of this pandemic has presented the entire world with the most complex set of challenges on the economic and public health fronts (Zhou, Chen, Zhan, Balamurugan & Thilak, 2021). India is no exception to this (Jha & Jha, 2020). One of the immediate effects of this situation is the Government of India providing several incentives and supportive measures to technology start-ups for generating innovative ideas and solutions to tackle COVID-19. Technology start-ups fall in the category of Micro, Small & Medium Enterprises (MSMEs) – a category which has been provided regulatory and economic support to start and sustain during this difficult situation. Start-up India, an initiative by the Government of India for handholding, funding support and incentives to start up ideas in India, took several measures to encourage innovative solutions to combat the pandemic. The details of these measures are enlisted in Table 5.

Table 5. Government of India Policy Measures for Technology Start-ups during COVID-19 in India. Source: Start-up India, 2021; Invest India, 2020

Funding Support	Regulatory Reforms and Economic Support	Open Challenges to Combat COVID-19	Mentoring and Visibility Support
• Grant Opportunities through Action COVID-19 Team (ACT) and US-India Science & Technology Endowment Fund (Covid Ignition Grants)	• Regulatory Reforms by Department for Promotion of Industry and Internal Trade (DPIIT)	• Department of Science & Technology: Centre for Augmenting War against COVID-19 Health Crisis (CAWACH)	• Sessions conducted by Start-up India with Start-up entrepreneurs, incubators, investors and mentors
• Debt & Returnable Grant Opportunities through Small Industries Development Board of India (SIDBI) SAFE, SIDBI SAFE PLUS, Department of Science & Technology (DST) CAWACH, SIDBI COVID-19 Start-up Assistance Scheme (CSAS)	• MSME Economic Package with new definition of MSMEs, emergency working capital facility, subordinate debt for stressed MSMEs, equity infusion for MSMEs	• MeitY: Innovation Challenge for creating Video Conferencing Solutions	• Investor engagement through talks with angel investors, venture capitalists, private equity funds, venture debt providers etc.
• Equity Funding through Omidyar Network India Rapid Response Funding and Bexley Advisors Covid-19 Action Fund (BACoAF)	• Business Immunity Platform by Invest India and partnership of Invest India with SIDBI to respond and resolve queries of MSMEs	• First Hub to address queries of start-ups - set up by Biotechnology Industry Research Assistance Council (BIRAC)	• Launch of the COVID-19 platform to fast-track register and list all the suppliers and their products that can be used to curb the pandemic by Government e Marketplace (GeM)
• A repository of resources for Indian start-ups solving challenges created by COVID-19 voluntarily supported by 91Springboard	• Fintech to be used to enhance transaction-based lending using the data generated by e-marketplace	• COVID-19 Innovations Deployment Accelerator by C-CAMP and T-HUB COVID-19 Innovation Challenge	• e-marketing linkage for MSMEs to be promoted to act as a replacement for trade fairs and exhibitions

3. LONG TERM IMPACT OF COVID-19 ON TECHNOLOGY STARTUPS AND TECHNOLOGY ENTREPRENEURSHIP IN INDIA

Start-ups and entrepreneurship face innumerable challenges that exist independent of a crisis like pandemic. Although several challenges are universal in nature, there are some which are specifically applicable to technology start-ups in India. Korreck (2019) highlighted five challenges for technology start-ups in India.

- The Indian population is very diverse and digitally divided. This provides an opportunity; but continues to be a barrier to growth.

- Technology start up founders are all techies by education and may lack the business acumen to build and scale a start-up.

- Lack of innovativeness of Indian buyers can create obstacles to acceptance for tech start-ups when taking the products to market.

- Up to recent times, start-ups were not considered attractive employers due to their inherent risk of failure – thus, attracting the best talent was a challenge.

- The regulatory environment in India is considered to be complex. India jumped 79 positions from 142nd (2014) to 63rd (2019) in 'World Bank's Ease of Doing Business Ranking 2020', however in the ease of starting a business in the country India still ranks 136th (World Bank, 2020).

Some of the challenges mentioned above will not be nullified altogether but their impact is likely to be reduced in the long run due to COVID-19. This pandemic can be termed as an external enabler of entrepreneurship (Davidsson, Recker & Briel, 2021). It has triggered a host of opportunities for businesses, technology entrepreneurship in particular. This paradigm shift is likely to transform the landscape for technology start-ups. The further discussion analyses the long-term impact of this global pandemic on technology entrepreneurship in India.

a. 'New Normal' and Large-Scale Digitalisation in India

There are extensive speculations that once the COVID-19 situation eases, customers will revert back to their pre-COVID-19 needs and behaviours and firms will revert back to old business models. However, experts indicate that the 'new normal' will stay and guide the businesses towards a new equilibrium to settle at. The 'new normal' is being embraced widely, and will continue in future (Seetharaman, 2020). This pandemic has forced digitalisation on the Indian population; which will have a significant long-term impact. Indians have embraced digitalisation and digital technologies in several ways - even in the rural areas.

COVID-19 transformed ways of interacting, consumption behaviour, and needs for Indians. Internet and digital adoption in India has accelerated. As of January 2021, India had 1.1 billion mobile connections, which is 79% of the total population; 624 million internet users, which comprise 45% of the total population and 448 million active social media users, which are 32.3% of the total population. Internet users in India increased by 47 million (8.2%) between 2020 and 2021(Statista, 2021). Such a large-scale digitalisation will provide a direct impetus to technology entrepreneurship in India.

This digitalisation is supported by India's growth dynamics and demographic characteristics. India is one of the fastest growing major economies of the world (fifth largest in 2019 and sixth largest in 2020) and is expected to be in the top 3 by 2030 (IBEF Report, 2021). In addition to this, it has the world's largest youth population, leading to rich demographic dividends. Economic growth and a large young population boost technology entrepreneurship further.

b. Long-term Consequences of COVID-19 in Specific Technology Sectors

Technologies that have evolved or grown as a result of this pandemic are likely to develop into novel and feasible solutions to several current and anticipated problems. These technologies will be adopted in the long run and will have a significant influence on our lives beyond COVID-19. These technologies existed even before the outbreak of COVID-19; but their applicability has increased during this pandemic. Brem, Viardot and Nylund (2021) classify these technologies into two categories:

- Technologies for saving life and improving health
- Technologies for improving quality of life

Table 6 and 7 discuss the long-term repercussions of these technologies on our lives. This, in turn, defines the long-term future of technology entrepreneurship also.

Table 6. Long-term Effects of Select Technologies Beyond COVID-19: Technologies for Saving Life and Improving Health

Primary Purpose of Technology	Type of Technology	Long-term Effect (Possibly Beyond COVID-19)
Saving Life and Improving Health	Flexible Manufacturing	• Redesign of medical equipment for faster and simpler manufacturing • Reinvent global supply chains for basic commodities like agriculture and energy to make them available in more geographically diverse areas
	Big Data Analytics	• Higher data monitoring and surveillance by companies and governments to prevent pandemics in future • Higher demand for cyber-security software and solutions to safeguard business and personal data against cyber-frauds
	3-D Printing	• Increased adoption of 3-D printing technology in health care, automotive, robotics etc. as 3-D printing becomes mainstream and moves from Business-to-Business (B2B) to Business-to-Consumer (B2C) markets
	Healthtech	• More use of healthcare features in smart gadgets • Increase in remote diagnostics, treatment and health monitoring • Development of virtual fitness studios and gyms

Source: Prepared by Author based on Brem, Viardot & Nylund (2021)

Table 7. Long-term Effects of Select Technologies Beyond COVID-19: Technologies for Improving Quality of Life

Primary Purpose of Technology	Type of Technology	Long-term Effect (Possibly Beyond COVID-19)
Improving Quality of Life	E-commerce and Logistics	• Higher market share of e-commerce in the total retail sector • Use of robots and drones to avoid human interaction
	Fintech	• Retaining the use of cashless payment modes • Higher use of mobile payment methods replacing plastic cards
	Edtech	• Increased market share of online learning programs compared to offline programs • Revising the content and pedagogy of teaching through online modes
	Video Conferencing	• 'Work From Home' model continues as it succeeds in being productive through advanced developments in video conferencing • Reduction in work-related travel • Spread of video conferencing technology among non-users
	E-gaming	• Virtual games develop professional leagues, sell merchandise, make high payments to star players in line with the offline games
	Internet Streaming	• With support from internet bandwidths, online news and home entertainment will gain traction

Source: Prepared by Author based on Brem, Viardot & Nylund (2021)

c. Sustainability Strategies for Technology Entrepreneurship in India

Technology start-ups have faced a high failure rate all over the world (Joshi & Achuthan, 2018). Only start-ups that overcome the initial challenges of funding and scalability can become successful (Bala Subrahmanya, 2015). Technology start-ups may be born out of disruptions such as COVID-19 but they will require specific strategies for long-run sustainability. "Sustainability is the cumulative effect of processes and products/services in an enterprise" – Karani & Mshenga, 2021. Several sustainability strategies can be analysed in the context of technology entrepreneurship.

- Shared Resources and Networking – Shared resources can improve resource access and reduce costs for start-ups. This is important at an initial stage when inflows could be limited. Collaboration and networking are important at an initial stage and social media networking could be the most cost-effective option for technology start-ups. With the rise in social media platforms, they provide a great asset to start-ups for networking. However, it can prove risky due to the freedom of information and speech associated with social media. A fabricated claim by competitors can destroy a start-up. When business grows for the start-up, the usefulness of social media networks supported by friends and family may reduce and wider networks may be required for scalability. The significance of continuous learning and experiments for gaining traction cannot be undermined in improving the sustainability of start-ups.

- Pivoting Business Models – Amid the pandemic, several technology start-ups (small and big) pivoted their business to suit the "new normal" and sustain themselves or adapt to changing consumer behaviour. This ability to pivot business models is highly significant for long-term sustainability. Several examples of pivoting strategies of technology start-ups are showcased in Figure 8.

Figure 8. Examples of Technology Start-ups Pivoting During COVID-19 in India

Bike-Taxi Startup Rapido	Event Management Startup Digital Jalebi	Digital streaming player Gaana
•Bengaluru-based startup had to initially suspend its operations in April 2020 temporarily due to the national lockdown • Later, the startup pivoted its model and began delivering essential items such as groceries and medicines to sustain its business and help people get their needed items at their doorstep, reducing the need for them to step out of their homes • The startup joined hands with Bigbasket, Big Bazaar, Spencer's Retail, and local authorities in Delhi and Bengaluru to help deliver basics	• Pre-COVID, this Bengaluru-based event management startup providing services related to venue planning, designing, infrastructure, technical support among many others • Understanding the accelerated digitisation in the event sector and the 'new normal', the founders pivoted to a web-based virtual event platform • The startup is focusing on recreating real-world experiences online from the comfort of homes - from any browser	•Had a large customer base of free users who had to listen to advertisements before the music played – during pre-COVID times • However, when advertisers cut their budgets due to the pandemic, this Indian startup made a lateral move. Gaana pivoted to offer original content in the form of podcast playlists by artists •It also ventured into localised content podcasts

Source: Prepared by author based on Ganguly (2020)

d. Resilience and Favourable Ecosystem - the key elements to Building and Sustaining Technology Entrepreneurship

The key to start-ups' long-term survival and prosperity lies in their resilience, their capability to absorb shocks and then rebound (Bigot & Germon, 2021). McKinsey's research in 2008 financial crisis differentiates a group of businesses that outperformed their competitors. They recovered much faster by redesigning business models and supply chains to reduce operating costs. "Decisions made during the crisis may well lead to an explosion of innovation and productivity to more resilient industries" – Bigot and Germon, 2021; pg 2.

COVID-19 has been 'a moment of truth' for many start-ups. Start-ups have not only realised the limitations, but also opportunities to save cost, be more efficient and resilient in the (post) COVID era. Technology entrepreneurs in India and across the world will have to learn/revise the art of resilience. This is very crucial to remain competitive in the long term (Jha, 2020).

Portuguez Castro and Gomez Germeno (2020) describe four levels of resilience for entrepreneurs – ranging from a micro to macro perspective. Figure 9 depicts the four levels of entrepreneurial resilience. All four levels of resilience are not directly related to entrepreneurs. Although entrepreneurial resilience generates from the entrepreneur, the other three levels of resilience need support though a favourable entrepreneurial ecosystem.

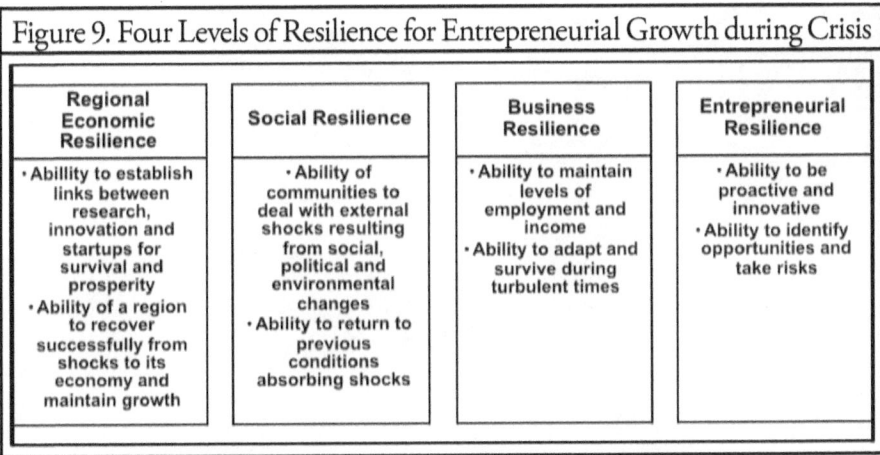

Figure 9. Four Levels of Resilience for Entrepreneurial Growth during Crisis

Regional Economic Resilience	Social Resilience	Business Resilience	Entrepreneurial Resilience
• Abillity to establish links between research, innovation and startups for survival and prosperity • Ability of a region to recover successfully from shocks to its economy and maintain growth	• Ability of communities to deal with external shocks resulting from social, political and environmental changes • Ability to return to previous conditions absorbing shocks	• Ability to maintain levels of employment and income • Ability to adapt and survive during turbulent times	• Ability to be proactive and innovative • Ability to identify opportunities and take risks

Source: Prepared by author based on Portuguez Castro & Gomez Germeno (2020)

Bala Subrahmanya (2017) lists 12 components of a robust technology entrepreneurial ecosystem. Table 8 throws light on the role and importance of these 12 components. COVID-19 has provided an impetus to technology entrepreneurship in India; however, the various stakeholders will have to focus on all these components for growth and sustainability of technology start-ups in India. India can take lessons from two often benchmarked technology entrepreneurship ecosystems in the world namely Silicon Valley and Israel.

Table 8. Role and Significance of Components of Technology Entrepreneurship

Component	Role	Component	Role
Markets	Early adopters, repeat clients, networks and Multi-National Corporations (MNCs)	Finance	Angel investors, private equity firms, venture capitalists, capital market and debt instruments
Human Resources	Labour, technical workforce and managerial talent	Education & Research	Institutions that generate technical and managerial skills, innovative thinking, and entrepreneurial abilities
Government Policies	Favourable regulations, tax incentives, venture capital, bankruptcy laws, property rights, labour laws, public research institutions	Large Businesses	As customers, sources of entrepreneurship, nurturers of start-ups through accelerators, investors, sources of technical and managerial workforce, technology providers and acquirers of start-ups
Mentors/Advisors	Technical and managerial advice for start-up creation, stability, growth and exit	Support Institutions	Accelerators, technology business incubators, soft infrastructure (e.g. lawyers and accountants), hard infrastructure (e.g. telecom, transportation, logistics)
Cultural Support	Tolerance for risk and failures, support for innovation and creativity, respect for wealth creation, higher social status for entrepreneurs	Media	Publicizing start up creations, its pre-requisites, support, failure consequences, and achievements
Entrepreneurship	At the heart of the ecosystem for birth, growth and exit of start-ups	Immigration of Talent	Sources of entrepreneurship, human resources, advisors, mentors, finance, support networks

Source: Bala Subrahmanya (2017); pg 49

4. A SNAPSHOT OF RESEARCH FROM SEVERAL NATIONS ON TECHNOLOGY STARTUPS AND TECHNOLOGY ENTREPRENEURSHIP DURING COVID-19

This section discusses how COVID-19 has impacted technology start-ups and technology entrepreneurship globally. It aims to provide an overview of the global research on impact of COVID-19 on technology start-ups and entrepreneurship. Globally businesses have identified and pursued technology entrepreneurial opportunities, tried to build up financial capabilities and rely on relational capabilities to overcome this crisis (Kuckertz, A. et. al., 2020). Several studies have pointed out to the growth of technology start-ups (and technology entrepreneurship, in turn) during the COVID-19 phase. Table 9 provides a snapshot of these studies. Studies from various nations suggest that COVID-19 has provided a huge impetus to technology start-ups and technology entrepreneurship, globally. However, policy decisions by governments will continue to be of utmost importance for sustainability and growth of these start-ups in future.

Table 9. Studies from Several Nations on Technology Start-ups & Technology Entrepreneurship during COVID-19

Sr. No.	Authors	Country Of Study	Methodology Of Study	Significant Findings
1.	Akpan, I. et al., 2020	USA & UK	Study of what will be the tech enablers for small business innovation	Identifies the technologies, evaluates disruptive software platforms, and strategies needed for creating and managing small business innovation during COVID-19
2.	Alves, J. et. al., 2020	Macau, China	Interview for data collection from six small local firms in Macau, China	As compared with large firms, new start-ups and small firms show high flexibility in their reactions to the crisis. Flexible HR strategies, increased product diversification and exploring new markets through technology were the core strategies
3.	Bakar, M. et. al., 2020	Malaysia	Qualitative study via document analysis approach using sources such as books, journal articles etc. on Islamic technopreneurship during COVID-19 era in Malaysia	Provides guidance to technologists, entrepreneurs, technology entrepreneurs as well as policy makers to present the concept, ideas and potential of Islamic Technopreneurship in a challenging era of COVID-19
4.	Dahlke, J. et al., 2021	Germany	Content Analysis of 707 innovation projects	Rapid-response COVID-19 innovations exhibit a diverse set of domains ranging from technological innovations to what may be described as frugal and social innovations.
5.	Ebersberger, B. & Kuckertz, A., 2021	Germany	Explore the impact of organisation type on innovation response time during COVID-19 by analysing data from a commercial innovation database	Technology start-ups collaborating with corporates and going for open innovation are likely to be more successful in the aftermath of COVID-19 crisis
6.	Kuckertz, A. et. al., 2020	Germany	Interviews with 16 start-up members (6 in the technology sector) asking about the adversity that start-ups faced during COVID-19 and their response mechanisms	Start-ups are successfully leveraging their available resources as a first response to the crisis, but their growth and innovation potential would depend on policy measures
7.	Maritz, A. et. al., 2020	Australia	Emergent enquiry narratives from leading Australian scholars, identifying entrepreneurial initiatives as a catalyst to new venture creation and growth during COVID-19	Insights associated with the entrepreneurial mindset, the multidimensional effects of resilience and entrepreneurship, entrepreneurship education, entrepreneurship enablers and the entrepreneurial ecosystem of Australia

8.	Markovic, et. al., 2021	Bosnia & Herzegovina	Qualitative data was collected from SMEs in Bosnia & Herzegovina	SMEs have embraced new collaborations with business customers and competitors, and developed a collaborative mindset aided by technology opposed to the traditionally competitive way of doing business in emerging markets
9.	Pastran, A., 2021	USA & Latin America	Study of successful examples of sustainable entrepreneurship in US and Latin America with focus on Smartly firm - how it helps fight economic crisis and changes in consumption	Public policy steps must be taken to generate long-term sustainability and scalable change after the pandemic and therefore, Smartly is actively engaged in lobbying initiatives to support the creation of a new sustainable legal framework
10.	Paul, J. et. al., 2020	China & India	Based on content analysis, discusses contemporary topics such as innovation, exports, foreign direct investment, technology, social capital, board independence as part of corporate governance and explores novel themes such as consumer behaviour in regard to luxury brands and women entrepreneurship in an emerging country context	There are several novel paradigms for new businesses in the context of China and India. A paradigm shift in diplomatic relations has taken place as an aftermath of COVID-19 in the world
11.	Polas, M. & Raju, V., 2021	Bangladesh	Electronic data from 127 SMEs of Bangladesh	Study of interplay between entrepreneurial opportunity recognition, opportunity development and opportunity exploitation with their entrepreneurial marketing decisions
12.	Scheidgen, K. et. al., 2021	Germany	Four rounds of data collection and four focus groups from 95 entrepreneurial activities in Germany	Entrepreneurs are proactive agents in alleviating the negative consequences of the COVID-19 crisis and digitalization is the key for entrepreneurs in this process
13.	Zhou, D. et. al., 2021	South Korea, China, India	Study of 1,000 participants from 3 countries to analyse the improvement in policy mechanisms for promotion of future technology businesses during COVID-19 pandemic	Governments contributed various policies to be followed to ensure sustainability of digital businesses during and after COVID-19

New rules of competition often appear during periods of transition. However, when the crisis subsides, as it will, although it may leave an economic crater behind, "true economic value once again becomes the final arbiter of business success" (Porter, 2001, pg. 65). Globally, COVID-19 has made it imperative for businesses to look for digital replacements or identify novel ways of delivering their products and service with minimal physical contact and safely.

These choices have presented opportunities for firms to be innovative in redesigning their existing products; designing alternative digital products and services; and/or rethink their product and service delivery channels and mechanisms; and to look for strategic positions and partners in the new ecosystem who can help them achieve these. In order to succeed in the new ecosystem, firms need to be agile, possess dynamic capabilities that can aid them in their adaptability to the changing times (Seetharaman, 2020). Although the immediate risks may disappear when COVID-19 situation improves, the opportunity presented for increasing degree of digitization in business firms remain. From a macro level perspective, technology start-ups and entrepreneurship across the world followed a similar pattern during COVID-19 as the one displayed in India.

5. CONCLUDING DISCUSSION

A recession changes the business model reducing costs and prices. On the other hand, pandemics create entirely new categories of business. Pandemics and recessions both prove to be accelerants to innovation. A 'once in a lifetime' event like COVID-19 has several immediate and long-term repercussions. This study provides several insights for technology entrepreneurship in India that arise from this global pandemic situation.

First, though digitalisation and adoption of digital technologies has accelerated, the importance of people management during crisis cannot be undermined. Ability to adapt, pivot and diversify has been crucial to success of technology start-ups in specific and all businesses in general during COVID-19. The fastest growth is witnessed and will continue in fintech, healthtech, edtech and SaaS sectors of technology start-ups.

Second, as COVID-19 becomes the 'new normal', the focus shifts from risk management to creative thinking for delivering products and services competitively. Technology has become a focal point of new business ideas as people become habitual of using more technology and practising social distancing (Paul, Menzies, Zutshi & Cai, 2020). Technology start up ideas that can be commercialised with minimum investments will be encouraged in India. This impact will continue in future as this pandemic has irrevocably changed the way businesses will compete over the next decade. Firms that choose to capitalize on these underlying changes will succeed in the long run.

Third, the way in which technology start-ups are impacted in the near future will have an impact on how entrepreneurship is perceived as a career choice in the long-term. By far, technology entrepreneurship was a privilege of the select few in specific ecosystems with the right kind of education, funding and networks. COVID-19 has provided the potential for democratizing technology entrepreneurship and creating novel entrepreneurial role models that Indians can more easily identify with. This could ultimately lower the threshold of entrepreneurship for many and encourage people to start their own businesses. The efforts to strengthen technology entrepreneurship ecosystem in India will call for joint action from all stakeholders.

References

Akpan, I., Soopramanien, D. and Kwak, D. (2020). Cutting-edge technologies for small business and innovation in the era of COVID-19 global health pandemic, *Journal of Small Business & Entrepreneurship*, DOI: https://www.tandfonline.com/doi/full/1 0.1080/08276331.2020.1799294

Alves, J., Lok, T., Luo, Y. and Hao, W. (2020). Crisis Management for Small Business during the COVID-19 Outbreak: Survival, Resilience and Renewal Strategies of Firms in Macau. Retrieved from DOI: http://dx.doi.org/10.21203/rs.3.rs-34541/v1

Amankwah-Amoah, J., Khan, Z. and Wood, G. (2021). COVID-19 and business failures: The paradoxes of experience, scale, and scope for theory and practice. *European Management Journal*, 39, 179-184.

Amin, K. Griffith, M. and Dsouza, D. (2020). Online Gaming during COVID-19 Pandemic in India: Strategies for Work-Life Balance. *International Journal of Mental Health and Addiction*, https://dx.doi.org/10.1007%2Fs11469-020-00358-1

Anupam, S. (2021). 6 Indian Healthtech Startups to Watch Out For in 2021. Retrieved from https://inc42.com/infocus/startup-watchlist-2021/startup-watchlist-6-indian-healthtech-startups-to-watch-out-for-in-2021/

Bakar, M., Bakar, A., Noor, A. and Mohamad, N. (2020). Islamic Technopreneurship in the Midst of COVID-19 Pandemic: A Malaysia Review. *PalArch's Journal of Archaeology of Egypt/Egyptology*, 17(2) (2020), 1-11. ISSN 1567-214X.

Bala Subrahmanya, M. H. (2015). New Generation Startups in India: What Lessons Can We Learn from the Past? *Economic and Political Weekly*, 50(12): 56–63.

Bala Subrahmanya, M. H. (2017). Comparing the Entrepreneurial Ecosystems for Technology Startups in Bangalore and Hyderabad, India. *Technology Innovation Management Review,* 7(7), 47-62.

Bhalla, K. (2020). 2020 In Review: How Indian Startups Backed The Fight Against COVID-19. Retrieved from https://inc42. com/infocus/year-end-review-2020/2020-in-review-how-indian-startups-backed-the-fight-against-covid-19/

Bhattacharya, A. (2020). For some Indian software startups, it's almost like the Covid-19 lockdown never happened. Retrieved from https://qz.com/india/1907751/how-indian-saas-startups-are-thriving-during-coronavirus-pandemic/

Bigot, G. and Germon, R. (2021). Resilience, digitalization, and CSR's three pillars to develop robust post-COVID MSMEs. *Journal of International Council for Small Business,* https://doi.org/10.1080/26437015.2020.1852061

Brannen, S., Ahmed, H. and Newton, H. (2020). Covid-19 reshapes the future. *Centre for Strategic and International Studies.* https://www.jstor.org/stable/resrep25198

Brem, A., Viardot, E. and Nylund, P. (2021). Implications of the coronavirus (COVID-19) outbreak for innovation: Which technologies will improve our lives? *Technological Forecasting and Social Change,* 163, 120451.

Dahlke, J., Bogner, K., Becker, M., Schlaile, M., Pyka, A. and Ebersberger, B. (2021). Crisis-driven innovation and fundamental human needs: A typological framework of rapid-response COVID-19 innovations. *Technological Forecasting and Social Change,* 169, 20799.

Dash, S. (2020). The Impact of IoT in Healthcare: Global Technological Change & The Roadmap to a Networked Architecture in India. *Journal of Indian Institute of Science,* 100(4), 773-785.

Davidsson, P., Recker, J. and Briel, F. (2021). COVID-19 as External Enabler of entrepreneurship practice and research. *Business Research Quarterly*, 1-10.

Ebersberger, B. and Kuckertz, A. (2021). Hop to it! The impact of organization type on innovation response time to the COVID-19 crisis. *Journal of Business Research*, 124, 126-135.

Eggers, F. (2020). Masters of disasters? challenges and opportunities for SMES in times of crisis. *Journal of Business Research*, 116, 199–208.

Ganguly, S. (2020). Here are the Top 5 Pivot and Persist stories about startups that changed their business models amidst COVID-19. Retrieved from https://ca.news.yahoo.com/review-2020-top-5-pivot-005000594.html

Godha, A. and Sharma, A. (2021). Edtech startups capitalising over e-learning market after COVId-19 hit distress in India: The Road Ahead. *The Online Journal of Distance Education and E-learning*, 9(1), 28-38.

Gupta, R., Jain, K., Kusre, A. and Momaya, K. (2015). *Technological Entrepreneurship Ecosystem in India: Findings from a Survey.* POMS 26th Annual Conference, Washington, DC, USA.

Hisrich, R., Peters, M. and Shepherd, D. (2017). *Entrepreneurship.* Mc-Graw Hill Education, New York. ISBN: 978-0-07-811284-3

IBEF Report 2021. Retrieved from https://www.ibef.org/economy/indian-economy-overview

Invest India. (2020). Entrepreneurship in India. Retrieved from https://www.investindia.gov.in/setting-up-business-in-india

Jha, A. and Jha, R. (2020). India's response to COVID-19 crisis. *The Indian Economy Journal*, 68(3), 341-351.

Jha, C. (2020). The Great Disruptive Transformation: The Impact of COVID-19 crisis on Innovative Startups in India. Doctoral Thesis retrieved from https://gupea.ub.gu.se/bitstream/2077/66823/1/gupea_2077_66823_1.pdf

Joshi, D. (2021). Role of Culture in Success of Global High-Tech Startup Businesses from India. In Thakkar, B. (Eds.) *Culture in Global Businesses – Addressing National and Organizational Challenges;* 133-182. Palgrave Macmillan, Springer International Publishing AG, Switzerland.

Joshi, D. and Achuthan, S. (2018). Leadership in Indian High-tech Start-ups: Lessons for Future. In Thakkar, B. (Eds.) *The Future of Leadership: Addressing Complex Global Issues;* 39-92. Palgrave Macmillan, Springer International Publishing AG, Switzerland.

Karani, C. and Mshenga, P. (2021). Steering the sustainability of entrepreneurial start-ups. *Journal of Global Entrepreneurship Research,* https://link.springer.com/article/10.1007/s40497-021-00279-w

Kaur, N. and Sahdev, S. (2020). Fighting COVID-19 with technology and innovation, evolving and advancing with technological possibilities. *International Journal of Advanced Research in Engineering & Technology,*11(7), 395-405.

Korreck, S. (2019). *The Indian startup ecosystem: Drivers, challenges and pillars of support. Observer Research Foundation,* Occasional Paper No. 21

Kuckertz, A., Brandle, L., Gaudig, A., Hinderer, S., Reyes, C., Prochotta, A. et. al., (2020). Startups in times of crisis – A rapid response to the COVID-19 pandemic. *Journal of Business Venturing Insights,* 13, e00169.

Madnani, D.; Fernandes, S. and Madnani, N. (2020). Analysing the impact of COVID-19 on over-the-top media platforms in India. *International Journal of Pervasive Computing and Communications,* 16(5), 457-475.

Maritz, A., Perenyi, A., Waal, G. and Buck, C. (2020). Entrepreneurship as the Unsung Hero during the Current COVID-19 Economic Crisis: Australian Perspectives. *Sustainability, 12*, 4612; https://www.mdpi.com/2071-1050/12/11/4612

Markovic, S., Koporcic, N., Arslangic-Kalajdzic, M., Kadic-Maglajlic, S., Bagherzadeh, M. and Islam, N. (2021). Business-to-business open innovation: COVID-19 lessons for small and medium-sized enterprises from emerging markets. *Technological Forecasting & Social Change,* 170, 120833.

Mittal, A. & Shah, S. (2021). Startup ecosystem breathes new life into India's Covid fight. Retrieved from https://economictimes.indiatimes.com/tech/startups/startup-ecosystem-breathes-new-life-into-indias-covid-fight/articleshow/82246612.cms

Mitter, S. (2021). One year of lockdown: 10 Indian startups that rode edtech's hockey stick curve in the pandemic. Retrieved from https://yourstory.com/2021/03/one-year-lockdown-indian-startups-edtech-hockey-stick-growth/amp

Narayanan, V. (2021). Covid is big stimulus for health tech startups. Retrieved from https://www.thehindubusinessline.com/info-tech/covid-is-big-stimulus-for-health-tech-start-ups/article34429314.ece

NASSCOM. (2020). Nasscom start-up pulse survey – ql 2020: Reviving the indian tech start-up engine during Covid 19. Retrieved from https://www.google.co.in/url?sa=t&rct=j&q=&esrc=s&source=web&cd=&ved=2ahUKEwiZ2ufwnaT2AhUAUWwGHZl5CGIQFnoECBcQAQ&url=https%3A%2F%2Fcommunity.nasscom.in%2Fcommunities%2Fproduct-startups%2Fnasscom-start-up-pulse-survey-ql-2020-reviving-the-indian-start-up-engine-during-covid-19.html&usg=AOvVaw0ze9Vxd5NEICCa7fTXBpfl

Pastran, A., Colli, E. and Poclaba, C. (2021) Sustainable entrepreneurship: A new way of doing business. *Journal of the International Council for Small Business,* 2(2), 147-158.

Paul, J., Menzies, J., Zutshi, A. and Cai, H. (2020). New and novel business paradigms in and from China and India. *European Business Review,* 32 (5), 785-800.

Polas, M. and Raju, V. (2021). Technology and Entrepreneurial Marketing Decisions During COVID-19. *Global Journal of Flexible Systems Management,* 22(2), 95-112.

Porter, M. (2001). Strategy and the internet. *Harvard Business Review,* 79(3), 62–78.

Portuguez Castro, M. and Gómez Zermeño, M.G. (2020). Being an entrepreneur post-COVID-19 – resilience in times of crisis: a systematic literature review. Journal of Entrepreneurship in Emerging Economies, Vol. ahead-of-print No. ahead-of-print. https://www.emerald.com/insight/content/doi/10.1108/JEEE-07-2020-0246/full/html

PTI (2021). India sees 60 percent rise in fintech deals amidst COVID-19; surpasses China, says report. Retrieved from https://yourstory.com/2021/02/india-surpasses-china-fintech-deals-upi-paytm-phonepe-google-pay/amp

Rakshit, S., Islam, N., Mondal, S., and Paul, T. (2021). Mobile apps for SME business sustainability during COVID-19 and onwards. *Journal of Business Research,* 135, 28-39.

Rao, P., Goyal, N., Kumar, S., Hassan, K. and Shahimi, S. (2021). Vulnerability of financial markets in India: The contagious effect of COVID-19. *Research in International Business and Finance,* 58, 101462.

Scheidgen, K., Gumusay, A., Gunzel-Jensen, F., Krlev, G. and Wolf, M. (2021). Crises and entrepreneurial opportunities: Digital social innovation in response to physical distancing. *Journal of Business Venturing Insights,* 15, e00222.

Seetharaman, P. (2020). Business models shifts: Impact of covid-19. *International Journal of Information Management,* 54, 102173.

Shah, S. (2020). 2020 year in review: Risk investors pour $9.3 billion into Indian startups despite Covid-19 woes. Retrieved from https://economictimes.indiatimes.com/tech/funding/risk-investors-pour-in-9-3-billion-in-2020-to-back-indian-startups-despite-covid-19-woes/articleshow/79981602.cms

Sheth, H. (2020). Podcast listening is growing in India: Spotify. Retrieved from https://www.thehindubusinessline.com/info-tech/podcast-listening-is-growing-in-india-spotify/article33295648.ece

Simo´n-Moya, V., Revuelto-Taboada, L., and Ribeiro-Soriano, D. (2016). Influence of economic crisis on new SME survival: Reality or fiction? *Entrepreneurship & Regional Development,* 28(1-2), 157–176.

Singh, M., Adebayo, S., Saini, M. and Singh, J. (2021). Indian government E-learning initiatives in response to COVID-19 crisis: A case study on online learning in Indian higher education system. *Education and Information Technologies,* https://link.springer.com/article/10.1007/s10639-021-10585-1

Sreenivasan, A. and Suresh, M. (2021), Modeling the enablers of sourcing risks faced by startups in COVID-19 era. *Journal of Global Operations and Strategic Sourcing,* Vol. ahead-of-print No. ahead-of-print. https://www.emerald.com/insight/content/doi/10.1108/JGOSS-12-2020-0070/full/html

Startup Genome, 2020. The Global Startup Ecosystem Report, 2020. Retrieved from https://startupgenome.com/report/gser2020

Startup India (2021). Retrieved from https://www.startupindia.gov.in/content/sih/en/covid-19_resource_section.html

Statista (2021). Digital population across India as of January 2021. Retrieved from https://www.statista.com/markets/424/internet/

Tripathi, S. and Brahma, M. (2017). Technology Entrepreneurship in Emerging Markets: An Exploration of Emerging Entrepreneurship Models Prevalent in India. *Technology Innovation Management Review*, 8(1), 24-32.

Venkataraman, S. and Shane, S. (2000). The promise of entrepreneurship as a field of research. *Academy of Management Review*, 25(1), 217–226.

Villaseca, D., Navio-Marco, J. and Gimeno, R. (2020). Money for female entrepreneurs does not grow on trees: start-ups' financing implications in times of COVID-19. *Journal of Entreprenurship in Emerging Economies, https://www.emerald.com/insight/content/doi/10.1108/JEEE-06-2020-0172/full/html*

WHO (2020, March 11). *WHO Director-General's opening remarks at the media briefing on COVID-19 - March 11, 2020.* Accessed July 18, 2020 from https://www.who.int/director-general/speeches/detail/who-director-general-s-opening-remarks-at-the-media-briefing-on-covid-19---11-march-2020

World Bank. (2020). Ease of doing business rankings. Retrieved from https://www.doingbusiness.org/en/rankings

Zhou, D., Chen, Z., Zhan, X., Balamurugan, S. and Thilak, D. (2021). Improved policy mechanisms for the promotion of future digital business economy during covid-19 pandemic. Electronic Commerce Research, https://link.springer.com/article/10.1007/s10660-021-09484-x

CHAPTER 6

Change Management Complexities during Pandemic Faced by Managers and Leaders

by Indranie Gurusamy Ram

Abstract

This chapter analyzes how various leaders across the globe managed the challenges during the pandemic. COVID-19, an unprecedented pandemic, left the human race in a state of disintegration. During a period of fear and uncertainty, without prior warnings, as was the case at the onset of COVID-19, the actions and leadership of decision-makers are crucial, in particular the change management strategies that are used to effect a successful outcome. The dilemma for decision-makers to choose between the lives of their citizens or to sustain the economy is examined and discussed. Assumptions regarding resources and healthcare systems were at the center of many of these dilemmas facing decision-makers. The complexity in reaching a solution regarding what to permit and what to prohibit seemed to be changing and becoming elusive as the virus continued to infect huge numbers of the population and spread rapidly. The importance of taking decisive actions to slow down the spread of the virus is discussed with emphasis on how effective the change management approaches were. The communication approach that leaders adopted with their citizens which was an integral component in creating trust and building confidence is analyzed. As the catastrophic reality of the pandemic became visible on the media, for many citizens, the only guidance and support they felt they had were their leaders.

Leaders felt the responsibility and the resources of leading their citizens out of the pandemic, were in their domain. How leaders handled the pressure and provided the relevant guidelines to their citizens is examined. Change management models currently being used in organizations will be presented and the complexity of using these models due to a lack of time is analyzed, taking into account the unique demands of the pandemic. The scientific community's dependency on funding and the ethical dimensions of how information was shared and how priorities within the scientific community were established are examined. The scientists realized the urgency to develop a vaccine, and this became a priority. The application of strategic collaboration and cooperation by the leaders and the scientific community are analyzed.

Keywords: Leadership, change management, challenges, decision making, resources, citizens, vaccinations, the impact of COVID-19

"Change is a phenomenon that occurs within communication"
Ford&Ford (1995)

1.0 Introduction

In this chapter, change management approaches used by global leaders and decision-makers in adopting unique and ground-breaking insights to reach the required outcome are analyzed. This analysis provides a framework of comprehensiveness and coherence showing how personal commitment, engagement, and leadership can transcend barriers and emerge with an implementable solution.

Change management is the development of a synthesis of processes which reflect the ways in which human beings behave and interact with each other from time to time in order to restore their sense of inhabiting a world of meaning and coexistence.

Global leaders and governments were faced with unprecedented challenges when COVID-19 spread globally. These challenges were complex enough for leaders to feel a sense of desperation when the change management approaches which they were accustomed to applying prior to COVID-19 seemed ineffective. Leaders were scrambling and looking for guidance from what other countries were doing.

Expert teams of scientists and medical professionals were working frantically together to solve, what seemed to be, an unsolvable puzzle. They were utilizing every opportunity that was presented to them to learn about the virus. They were observing the behavior of the virus, conducting empirically based research on sick patients in the hospitals, and performing autopsies on those who had died from COVID-19. The scientists were collectively working on the genome sequence of the virus to develop an efficacious vaccine. The right type of reforms needed to be made expediently.

Leaders and decision-makers were confronted with the challenging problem of dealing with an environment rife with turmoil, disintegration, unbalanced, and disorderly citizens plagued by anxiety, nightmares, fears, uncertainty, and lack of trust. There were galactic shifts in the world and it seemed like the balance was lost. The feeling among people could be compared to the aftermath of a nuclear power explosion. Reality had changed in an instant. Lifton (1983) argues that vivid end-of-the-world imagery involves "an anticipatory imagination capable of sensitivity to a trend of events which other people have become numb to." It is interesting that many communities when they become numb with fear, also become inactive in a situation which potentially can have devastating consequences for their survival.

Lifton (1983) coined the phrase *psychic numbing* Lifton stated that when survivors of the first atomic bomb dropped on a human population in Hiroshima were interviewed they often described their minds as kind of shutting. He called that psychic numbing. Lifton says, "It can be adaptive," helping people cope in some situations. In their cases, he says it was a defense mechanism to get through the experience.

Professor Lifton's findings are very relevant to the psychological states, I believe, of people during the pandemic. Their anxiety, and their fear of the unknown, has left them in a state of psychic numbing, which I also believe is a coping mechanism as the virus spreads and mutations are appearing.

2.0 Origins of COVID-19

There is still a great deal of ambiguity regarding the origins of COVID-19. The global community understands that it emanated from Wuhan in Hubei Province in China. The virus first demonstrated its existence in Wuhan in November/December 2019 and only reached other countries a few months later supposedly from people who travelled out of Wuhan. There were delays in reporting from Wuhan because they did not realize they were facing a catastrophic pandemic. If the contagion was restricted to Wuhan, the rest of the world would have been saved. Although they imposed a lockdown, some travelers, especially businesspeople from other countries left, and they apparently took the virus with them. South Africa's first case of coronavirus was in March 2020, a tourist who had returned from Italy. Subsequently the South African National Health Department started a track and trace system to restrict the spread of the virus. All the people on the plane with that individual were contacted and informed they had been in contact with someone who had the coronavirus, and they needed to self-isolate. This approach was working, and the numbers were initially very low in South Africa. Problems and challenges arose when all the people that were in contact with an infected person could not be traced or informed and unwittingly they were spreading the virus.

3.0 What Is Change Management?

Change management is a complex process, not just a linear process following a set number of steps or stages in a particular sequence. There are at various stages of the fast-changing, uncertain, dynamic, and turbulent process overlaps and backward and forward interplays as the process evolves and learning is tested and implemented. With COVID-19, there needs to be continuous monitoring of the situation and statistics provide vital feedback, so appropriate action can be taken as soon as a spike is detected. It is an iterative process. The model is cyclical and the change is ongoing.

In 2011, Kotter acknowledged the limitations of change management in the context of the term change leadership. It's trying to make sure change is done efficiently in the sense of you don't go over budget—another control piece.

Kotter (2011) in his book *Leading Change* defines management and leadership as "leadership defines what the future should look like, aligns people with that vision, and inspires them to make it happen despite the obstacles."

Harvey and Brown (2001) in a similar vein state the following, "In a turbulent and changing environment, managers are concerned not only with managing organizations as they exist in the present time but also with changes to meet future conditions. Change programs do not happen accidentally. Instead, they are initiated with a specific purpose and require some form of leadership to function properly."

Harvey and Brown (2001) state, "Change is avalanching down upon our heads and most people are utterly unprepared to cope with it. Organizations are changing and will continue to do so in order to survive in this complex environment."

3.1 Relationship between Choice and Change Management

Change and making the choices that enable us to survive is the very substance of our lives. The element of personal responsibility is demonstrated in the choices one makes. In the moment of making a decision when change needs to be adopted, we are making a choice. We may also feel that we have no choice at all because the change has to be made at a crucial juncture, or the consequences can be devastating. This is the kind of demanding and stressful environment leaders found they were in when the pandemic was ravaging their citizens. The changes thrust onto the world when the pandemic became widespread are radical if not catastrophic. There are no comparisons post World War II that required the strategic, decisive, and scientific interventions to save human lives that leaders were faced with during the pandemic. This was a time that required and demanded the creation of new ways of thinking, new blueprints of working together, and new styles of international leadership. On a very practical and urgent level, it required the creation of a workable worldwide infrastructure of trusting relationships and functional solutions. Sharing information and expertise became both critical and urgent. The advent of COVID-19 required leaders and citizens to think more deeply about their future and the changes they need to make to survive.

The WHO (World Health Organization) became the conductor of an orchestra of countries walking in the dark and looking for any light at the end of the tunnel. The creation of an efficacious vaccination was envisioned as the light at the end of the tunnel. Decision-makers and leaders globally had to create a set of realistic priorities about what needed to be done in a systematic, logical, and organized way. The puzzle which presented itself as COVID-19 needed to be solved and an approach the leaders adopted was to work collaboratively and to focus on the healthcare systems. Assumptions regarding resources especially of healthcare systems were at the center of many of these dilemmas facing decision-makers. Many countries believed their hospitals, and healthcare workers were ill-equipped to deal with a pandemic. There was a shortage of beds, staff, personal protective equipment (PPE) for staff to wear, medication, ventilators, and a multitude of other health-related requirements. It became a frenzy to equip hospitals with relevant infrastructure and equipment. Current literature abounds with information around the management of COVID-19 challenges, as well as patients with co-morbidities especially diabetes and cardiac conditions (see Adams and Walls 2020; Koliaki et al. 2020; Sommer et al. 2020).

3.2 Decision-Making Complexities

Dilemmas facing leaders are the following:

- choice between lives of citizens and livelihoods
- assumptions regarding resources and healthcare systems
- what to permit and what to prohibit seemed to be changing
- what guidelines to give to citizens
- how and what information needs to be shared
- how to develop long-term countermeasures

The complexity in reaching a solution regarding what to permit and what to prohibit seemed to be changing and becoming elusive as the virus continued to infect huge numbers of the population and spread rapidly. According to a joint statement made by International Labor Organizations (ILO), Food and Agriculture Organization of the United Nations (FAO), International Fund for Agricultural Development (IFAD), and World Health Organization (WHO) on October 13, 2020, "The economic and social disruption caused by the pandemic is devastating: tens of millions of people are at risk of falling into extreme poverty, while the number of undernourished people, currently estimated nearly 690 million, could increase by up to 132 million by the end of the year. Millions of enterprises face an existential threat. Nearly half of the world's 3.3 billion global workforce is at risk of losing their livelihoods. Without the means to earn an income during lockdowns, many are unable to feed themselves and their families. In the COVID-19 crisis food security, public health, and employment and labor issues, in particular workers' health and safety converge." Leaders in their decision-making processes had to take into account the fear of COVID-19 lingering and companies not surviving long periods of lockdowns. What impact would this have on the economy? Would it be possible for businesses to reinvent themselves? During a period of fear and uncertainty without prior warnings as was the case at the onset of COVID-19, the actions and leadership of decision-makers are crucial, in particular the change management strategies that are used to effect a successful outcome. Miller (2018) states, "The use of tacit knowledge and educated judgment relate to intuitive decision making which has been emphasized in crisis situations." Boin (2005) has stated, after a review of crisis research, that a crisis can destabilize the organization and its workers.

3.3 How Leaders Handled the Pressure in Providing Guidelines?

The immediacy leaders faced of having to make decisions and the lack of preparedness on the part of leadership when WHO announced that the world was facing a pandemic was an unknown and unquantifiable global phenomenon. Many world leaders were faced with choices and decisions which were untested and the hesitancy was palpable. If there was a time in the history of humanity when time was running against humanity, it was at the outbreak of the pandemic. Decisiveness was crucial but how leaders handled this pressure and provided the relevant guidelines to their citizens became crucial to upholding the structures that society had become accustomed to. Leaders need to find a way to assuage people's fears. We should not underestimate the degree of disturbance in the average person. They are clearly aware and deeply concerned about COVID-19, and it is constantly in their minds. The solutions must be perceived to be scientifically effective and something the ordinary person is capable of doing.

There were some leaders who delayed their decision-making to see what approaches would work in other countries. If one has to define the change management approach that was adopted by decision-makers and leaders regarding COVID-19, one would say it was an approach of "learn what worked in other countries and improve on their errors." This was the only resource available because any amount of theory that was written on change management usually would require planning, consultation, and time. They had to adopt a reactive approach and act with the most urgent expediency the human race had experienced. This approach in hindsight only exacerbated the problem. The longer it took leaders to implement a total lockdown, which now, a year and a half later can be seen to have been a crucial decision, and the leaders' indecision led to a greater spread of the virus. Leaders were confronted with the problem and challenge of how to sustain and maintain equilibrium in the midst of turbulence. Lockdowns and forced quarantines on a scale not seen before were enforced, different methods and procedures being applied by different countries.

The business sector did not realize the urgency of closing their businesses. COVID-19 put unprecedented challenges on small businesses, many of the small businesses did not survive the lockdowns, and many had to dismiss their staff and close. The pandemic had a devastating impact on the economy and businesses globally. For example, the oil prices went down, and it became very difficult for governments to sustain their economies. Many global leaders tried to stimulate their economies by introducing stimulus packages and slashing spending. Stimulus packages helped many small businesses and people who lost their jobs. Banks reduced interest rates, which affected the citizens' investments and pensions.

3.4 The Importance of Effective Communication

Leaders have a responsibility to communicate with their people, whether it is good or bad news. In a crisis situation, it makes a difference, and people rally around this communication for the actions they will take. Leaders, during a crisis, are a repository to the people and the architects of society. Hearing regularly from team leaders, taking perspective, and ensuring the well-being of those impacted by the pandemic are one of the core responsibilities of the leaders at the time of a pandemic and business lockdown. Wooten and James (2008), "By sharpening their emotional quotient, leaders would have a more empathetic response to the needs of their employees."

Although scientists are being admonished to join in the battle against misinformation (Fleming 2020; Thorp 2020), I believe it is the responsibility of leadership to lead by example and follow the protocols given by scientists based on empirical evidence and statistics and communicate accurate guidelines and valid information regularly to their citizens. Benabou, Falk, and Tirole's (2018) views are "strong leadership is so important and crucial during these turbulent and uncertain times and they have a powerful overall effect on what people believe and will do, because leaders can affect individuals' beliefs about the morality of costly actions." Economist Herbert Simon's (1996) view that "everyone designs who devises courses of action aimed at changing existing situations into preferred ones" is a useful starting point for thinking about intentional change.

4.0 Change Management Models

There are various change management models currently being used in organizations but for the purposes of this chapter, and in light of COVID-19, there is a complexity and challenge during a pandemic of using these models effectively due to a lack of time in reaching a workable solution.

One of the earliest models of planned change was Kurt Lewin's (1951) three-step model of *unfreezing*, actively changing, and *refreezing*.

Kotter's eight-step model of change to transform an organization can be listed as follows:

- establishing a sense of urgency
- forming a powerful guiding coalition
- creating a vision
- communicating the vision
- empowering others to act on the vision
- planning for and creating short-term wins
- consolidating improvements and producing still more changes
- institutionalizing new approaches

The Kubler-Ross change curve model provides seven stages on a curve. I have not included the diagram but just listed the stages as follows:

- shock—surprise or shock at the event
- denial—disbelief looking for evidence that it isn't true.
- frustration—recognition that things are different, sometimes angry
- depression—low mood, lacking energy
- experiment—initial engagement with the new situation

- decision—learning how to work in a new situation, feeling more positive
- integration—changes integrated, a renewed individual.

The SCARF model Rock (2008) is as follows:

S—status is about relative importance to others;

C—certainty concerns being able to predict the future;

A—autonomy provides a sense of control over events;

R—relatedness is a sense of safety with others;

F—fairness is a perception of fair exchanges between people.

This model is a useful way of understanding people's emotions.

4.1 Citizen's Perceptions

Besides having a capacity for reflective thought, the human person has a strong biological drive to live. We can describe a human being as having an instinct for life or an instinct for survival.

According to Aristotle, "The function of any living thing is to live." Aristotle says the best way of life is one in which each of us seeks to fit our feelings and desires into some coherent pattern. The scientists and leaders through empirical evidence were progressively cultivating their insights into how best to stop and defeat the virus, and by doing this, to use Aristotle's thinking, they were searching for *patterns*. They were making a concerted and sincere effort to allow human beings to live. The best guideline to follow according to Aristotle is to avoid extremes in our conduct or feelings.

Sometimes we have to do things or follow rules because we have to do them because we are under an obligation to do them like wearing a mask or not wearing a mask. The thinking and expertise required to find solutions and know the type of changes that were needed to control the spread of the virus seemed initially to be beyond our finite intelligibility of a virus that seemed, under thorough analysis to be one of the most complex structures, that scientists have seen. There was no complete picture of the potential harm this virus can cause to citizens, scientists, and leaders.

If one analyzes the decision by the scientists for everyone to wear a mask, practice social distancing, and wash hands with soap, these decisions are in keeping with, in my thinking, Kantian philosophy of the categorical imperative. According to Kant, a categorical imperative is a command of the form "you should do this" or "you ought not to do that." It is a genuine moral command that says what we must do regardless of whether we want to do it.

The scientists and lawmakers and leaders similarly believed they were acting on ethically and morally sound principles in making the wearing of masks, social distancing, and the washing of hands with soap and water, a universal rule because they believed it was the right thing to do, and by empirical evidence, these actions saved lives and prevented the virus from spreading.

The leaders and scientists were being optimistic that people will listen and follow the rules. Many conflicts arose and vast numbers of citizens believed their human rights were being suppressed and a considerable number of people broke the rules, which led to more infections. Some countries experienced rioting; people started marching and refusing to wear masks or adhere to the rules. This dissidence needed to be controlled and stemmed if any progress was going to be made to overcome the spread of the virus and reduce the daily death rate.

Sometimes rights need to be exercised in ways that might bring *unhappiness* depending on the urgency of the situation. To wear a mask and practice social distancing is also a matter of personal commitment and choice of the most abiding and significant sort, protecting your fellow human beings from infection. There was a need amongst communities to build confidence, to trust wearing a mask and going in public where there were other people. Social distancing needed to be enforced because scientists had calculated the virus cannot travel more than a certain distance if an infected person sneezed or coughed. Scientists believed if everyone wore a mask, practiced social distancing, washed hands with soap and water, practiced self-isolation, agreed to quarantine, governments enforced testing and tracing, and imposed lockdowns, the spread of the virus could be controlled.

There needed to be a change of mindset among citizens for survival. What kind of psychological scars will be created and are there resources to deal with the feelings of deep depression and hopelessness being felt by humanity as a whole. In some aspects, there was doubt in the mind of citizens because they did not really know and understand the cause of the virus; many believed it was God's punishment being cast on humanity, and to these believers, probably there were no scientific solutions so the route of following the dictates of science to them seemed inappropriate. To these believers, the answers lay in prayer and redemption by humanity. It can be stated for any individual to follow rules and regulations as laid out even by leaders, a prerequisite is trust. People became very suspicious of everything they were told or heard, some believed these were government conspiracies. Leaders had to exercise an extreme level of precaution when addressing their citizens. It was an environment where the need for cooperation, security and protection, and defense of the lives of the citizens are to be at the forefront of how leaders interacted with their citizens. Leaders need to be cognizant of the interplay between different elements during a crisis and how to manage those elements. Working with stakeholders requires cooperation and trust, and within communities, there are various levels of stakeholders, businesspeople, people from various professions, and various socioeconomic groups.

When change is going to be implemented, decision-makers need to do a force-field analysis of which groups of people are the helping forces and which groups of people constitute the hindering forces. Theory and experience suggest it is prudent to try to increase the helping forces and work on strategies of getting the participation of the hindering forces. The hindering forces can prove to be problematic if not handled appropriately. The control and management of the virus are dependent on human behavior and their perceptions; it was important they got the correct messages and modified their behavior. Peoples' experiences and interpretations of the pandemic differed dramatically from one day to the next depending on the daily death rate and the progress scientists were making in developing an efficacious vaccine. For many citizens, experience and empirical evidence played an important role regarding their perceptions of the virus.

Once people were vaccinated, it became easier for them to revert to old ways of doing things; how to refreeze and sustain or reinforce the changed behavior in accordance with the third stage of Lewin's model was a challenge. Questions around ongoing support, for example, awareness campaigns or even rewards were being posed by global leaders.

4.2 Resistance to Change

When you start discussing change, you are requesting those who are involved in the change process to leave their comfort zone to enter the unknown and use their energy on something new and different. Unless there is strong belief and acceptance of the change, you might encounter resistance. Resistance is a barrier, a hurdle preventing someone from moving forward with the proposed change. In most change situations, if the whole situation is not understood and the need for change has not been discussed and explained, there is a void in the mind of the citizens and leads to circular fabrications of future outcomes. This doubt or uncertainty can have an impact on productivity and peace of mind. It is important when leaders are discussing COVID-19 with their communities they keep their focus on ongoing research and development to overcome the pandemic and to instill their citizens with confidence and motivate them to remain calm and positive. In the throes of this pandemic, people had to find the strength within themselves to survive and guard their lives and the lives of their families. To change perceptions and attitudes is extremely complex unless the outcome is known, and there are high levels of trust. The relationship of irrational thoughts, fear, uncertainty, and suspicion, and the perceived impact of this pandemic set in motion a perceived resistance to change.

Oreg (2003) studied personality characteristics that predisposed individuals toward resisting change. Factors examined which influence a predisposition toward resistance included an inclination to seek routines, negative reactions to announcements of change, a short-term focus, and a rigid or dogmatic point of view. Furst and Cable (2008) examined how resistance to organizational change is related to a supervisor's managerial tactics and the employee's relationship with that supervisor. Weaker relationships led to greater resistance and stronger relationships showed less resistance.

Citizens' resistance to change became very complex when they demonstrated hesitancy to be vaccinated. This became very difficult to control when the mutations of the virus were spreading rampantly. It was evident that those who became very ill and required hospitalization were mainly among the unvaccinated.

5.0 Role of Scientists and Healthcare Workers

The real heroes and heroines of COVID-19 are the healthcare workers and the scientists. The dedication and loyalty they showed to the patients and the long hours of grueling, hard work they performed was an admirable feat. The scientific community worked endlessly to accomplish the creation of vaccines in under a year. The development of other vaccines, for example, measles, polio, smallpox, etc., took a minimum twelve years with the various levels of testing. The scientists knew they did not have the time to do that. Once they knew the composition or genome sequence of the virus, they started their controlled tests and within a year various vaccines emerged. The list ofCOVID-19 vaccines as listed by WHO are Pfizer/BioNTech Comirnaty, SII/Covishield and AstraZeneca/AZD1222, Janssen/Ad26. COV2.S developed by Johnson and Johnson, Moderna COVID-19, Sinopharm produced by Beijing Bio-Institute of Biological Products Co Ltd, Sinovac-CoronaVac.

Scientists around the world depend on one another to interpret information and data accurately and fairly and share their insights widely. At the beginning of the pandemic, no one had the keys to open the doors to guide the next step in the process, but through the diligent effort of the health workers, scientists, and thinkers working together effectively, some keys were being found. A newfound reality of hope and interdependence was emerging that we were in this together, and all countries needed to help each other to be able to see the next day.

How to fathom something which was an invisible intruder was baffling and confusing to many scientists primarily because they could not initially see the whole picture of how the virus was behaving and did not know how devastating the consequences of delaying taking actions to keep people apart were. Every day that the scientific community battled, trying to figure what the virus's constituent components were, resulted in an exponential rampant spread of the virus among people and loss of life.

On July 1, 2020, Tiffanie Wen in her article "What makes people stop caring" states (Wen 2020), "The death of an individual can have a powerful effect on our emotions, but as numbers rise so does our indifference." In the same article, Tiffanie Wen continues: to state, "Even now we can see the same strange process happening as the worldwide death toll due to coronavirus rises. The number of lives claimed by the virus has already exceeded 400,000 and more than seven million cases have been recorded in 200 countries. Each death is a tragedy played out on an individual level, with a family left shocked and bereaved. But as we zoom out, can anyone really wrap their head around such large numbers?"

5.1 Effects of Lockdowns

The socioeconomic disparities in the world were already there, prior to COVID-19, but with the decision to enforce total lockdowns that many countries were forced into, those disparities became very pronounced.

South Africa, a country with one of the greatest divides between the rich and the poor globally, provided food parcels to the poor, but for how long could this be sustained? For many citizens in South Africa, the effects of long periods of lockdowns, unemployment, and corruption resulted in riots and looting by the poorer communities. It was sad and traumatizing to witness the scenes of looting and destruction as they were aired on national TV in South Africa and around the world. To live in a country where change, especially for the poor, happens at a slow and almost nonproductive pace can be dehumanizing and depressing. Although in the wealthier suburbs, the high standard and quality of life of some citizens are luxurious. South Africa is the tragic story of a country with some of the best mineral resources in the world and other natural resources, but the poverty-stricken lives of the masses of poor citizens do not reflect this. Freedom as the world perceives the people of South Africa to have accomplished is a sorry tale, and those living in the country are aware of this. COVID- 19 is really a great travesty for the poor, in particular, because prior to COVID-19, they lived on a day-to-day accrual of food and other things as they scavenged around, but now with the lockdowns, they cannot do that.

After the initial lockdowns were imposed and many approaches that were adopted by global leaders seemed to have been effective in reducing the number of people infected with the virus and the daily death rates were being reduced, a roadmap of how to lift the lockdown was implemented in the UK and other countries. There needed to be a cautious and careful step-by-step easing of the lockdown. Things that were being analyzed and monitored were how effective are the vaccines, did hospitalizations drop, was there a drop in the daily death rate, variations of the virus, and are there any new mutations?

5.2 Climate Change

Our world and planet is in a state of disintegration. Besides COVID-19, the effects of climate change have caused widespread fires, flooding, hurricanes, and the kind of devastation globally, which the human race has not been exposed to prior to the present and on such a scale.

As I am writing this chapter, the devastating and catastrophic effects of climate change and greenhouse gas emissions are ravaging Canada, Peru, Greece, and USA. Loss of property and life as a consequence of higher-than-normal temperatures for human beings to tolerate has caused raging infernos; this is all happening in the midst of the pandemic. People had to be evacuated, and firefighters are risking their lives.

Leaders at the Toronto Conference on the Changing Atmosphere established in 1988, placed climate change on the agenda of states. The core institutions of global climate governance, the Intergovernmental Panel on Climate change (IPCC) and the United Nations Framework Convention on Climate Change (UNFCCC) were established after the Toronto conference.

There are many conferences being held remotely on future plans to reduce the impact of climate change and many agreements being signed for actions to be taken for countries to comply.

According to Bentley B. Allan (2017), "Climate change and environmental degradation have pushed many people and landscapes beyond thresholds of resilience."

Ram, K. (2021) articulated this aspect very succinctly, "The desirable aspects of resilience, robustness, sustainability, and adaptive capacity have been empirically derived as traits of complex organizations capable of withstanding severe environmental perturbations such as viral pandemics, climate change and global warming."

5.3 Impact of COVID-19

The reaction to COVID-19 and the impact it had on the free movement people around the world have been experiencing show us how vulnerable the human race can be. Movement is essential in a global environment, and human beings have, prior to COVID-19, been functioning with relative ease globally. For vast numbers of people globally, the reality of what isolation and distancing really require and demand can become very disturbing even frightening when they realize they might not see their loved ones for lengthy periods. During the pandemic, the world paused and life as everyone knew and understood it to be, had changed fundamentally. There was a new and uncertain normal, which instilled fear and uncertainty in the minds of people as the numbers that were hospitalized and died went up at an alarming rate. The rapid increase in the daily death rate, firstly in Italy and thereafter in neighboring countries, instilled fear and panic in the minds of those who were watching and listening to the spread of the news globally.

There are now new norms of behavior, new fears, and new adjustments to behavior, especially for businesses. The tragedy of how small businesses suffered because of COVID-19 was seen in every country globally. In various sectors during the period of lockdowns, people lost their jobs. Hospitality, entertainment, and the aviation industries were the hardest hit.

Global leaders were already, in early 2019, dealing with high levels of unemployment and poverty, but when the COVID-19 virus reared its ugly head in early 2020, they were paralyzed into the realization that an already bleak global economic situation is going to get even worse. It became apparent to global leaders after observing and discussing how Wuhan and then Italy contained the rapid spread of the virus by enforcing lockdowns that they would have to adopt the same measures. This decision was not an easy one to make. If we analyze the complexity of a total lockdown, which people around the world were not accustomed to, and the economic, psychological, and a multitude of other problems that could emerge, it was one of the most difficult decisions global leaders had to make. Many global leaders chose to initially institute a partial lockdown, keeping essential services and businesses open.

A UNDP report stated, "The COVID-19 pandemic went from a direct health emergency to a systemic crisis affecting people's lives in multiple ways. COVID-19 impacts have been unprecedented because of its evolution from a health shock to a social and economic crisis."

COVID-19 created an environment rife with vulnerabilities. The pandemic exacerbated disparities between economic groups. The barriers that existed on the socioeconomic level among different people were more pronounced and accentuated.

Testing the impact and spread of the virus by enforcing partial lockdowns demonstrated to global leaders that this virus was a resilient virus, the numbers of people being infected with the virus continued to rise, and the daily death rate continued going up. This was a huge dilemma for global leaders and citizens as well, and there were no easy solutions. While global leaders were fighting this existential dilemma, teams of scientists around the globe were busy working on the development of vaccines. It became a global trend on every TV channel to start their broadcasts showing the previous days COVID-19 statistics. These statistics would be analyzed and aired before any other news. People were glued to their TV stations, listening and hoping to hear there was a breakthrough, and the scientists had developed an effective and efficacious vaccine. The only real hope for the survival of the human race was in the hands of scientists developing vaccines. The scenes shown on the TV of empty streets and people wearing personal protective equipment (PPEs), spraying sanitizers on surfaces, seemed to those watching, like an alternate reality, a movie set. Widespread meetings and brainstorming sessions were being conducted via Zoom, Skype, and other technological means of communicating. The people of the globe were using technology to communicate while any form of personal interaction was restricted. People were wearing masks, which became mandatory in many countries; they were told to wash their hands with soap and water and practice social distancing. The new rules took a long while for citizens to get used to. There were groups of people globally, who refused to comply and were suspicious of all forms of guidance and instructions on how to keep safe and stay healthy. The changes for them had not really reached a point within themselves to quickly adapt to a change which was well thought out and could save lives. For vast numbers of citizens, facts have to be verifiable to be believed, and everything regarding the pandemic was crisis management and reactive and this uncertainty in the minds of many citizens caused doubt and created panic. There was also a great deal of fake information and misinformation that was circling around on multiple social media platforms creating additional panic and confusion.

Initially the perception was this virus will not be around for too long and that thought kept people full of hope, but as the months rolled on and after 18 months, the virus is still with us and there are mutations of the virus; people are now fatigued and some of their initial adherence to stringent rule-based norms and behavior is starting to wane. When fatigue sets in, mistakes start happening, people become less focused and drop their guard, which in the context of how the virus and the mutations of the virus spread, is extremely dangerous. The initial virus was spread as a beta variant. This mutated and a new coronavirus, the delta variant, which spread more rapidly and was more deadly than the initial beta variant, emerged. As scientists are examining the blood samples of the victims of COVID-19, they are discovering the mutations of the virus and its resilience, which although people are vaccinated, with the new mutations spreading rapidly, humanity is still at risk from COVID-19.

Global organizations requested their staff to work from home during the lockdown. There were certain categories of jobs that enabled people to work from home, but for other hands-on and non-technology-related jobs, this proved to be virtually impossible to do and sustain during a lockdown.

As Kotler (1995) states, "Building new organizations that will prosper in the new climate requires great change. Incremental adjustments are insufficient . . . The key force behind successful transformation is always leadership."

Once people understand why there is a need for change, they are not so resistant to the idea of change. This Lewin explains happens during the *unfreezing* stage. Kohlis (2020) reported that "how you treat your employees will be remembered for years to come."

6.0 Conclusion

Leaders can be susceptible to psychological forces in times of crisis that would distract them from their roles as decision-makers. A broader analysis of change, if undertaken with the right ideals, should be expressive of human ideals, desires, hopes, attitudes, and intentions. The meaning and significance of creative activity are transformative and lead to greater awareness and participation in the change management process. Despite all the scientific progress to date, in the medical and technological fields, an invisible virus has baffled the human race. The modern world is witnessing the catastrophic consequences of disharmonious living.

We should use education and knowledge not as a means to prosperity and power of the individual and the state but as the process by which we may realize our potential as human beings.

Ram, I. G (2020) states, "Our contemporary ("materialistically") minded society, obviously, does not yet provide the solutions, but what prospects of human survival there are depend a great deal on the increase of the applicable behavior and attributes of accountable and responsible decision-makers, in particular a transparent and honest approach by governments, to resolving problems in an ethical manner for the benefit of the greater many."

For many the way to the future lies in a new synthesis of the rational, emotional, and ethical in a truly integrated vision which can animate all areas of human endeavor. The human race collectively should not, in the future, wait for a pandemic to realize, we all need to come together and work in a coherent and compatible system with the environment and nature so as to realize our meaningful existence and help future generations prevail against forces that menace the survival of humans and other species on our beautiful planet. In the course of this chapter, I have shown that authentic and successful leadership is possible if there is an understanding and collaboration of our common humanity, and leaders can provide a sense of direction, happiness, and provide a basis of hope for their citizens. This vision of a completed humanity in the midst of COVID-19, which is fraught with images that symbolize a fragmentation of existence and human life, is surely one of the most challenging tasks facing leaders and decision-makers.

The future vision of leaders and decision-makers needs to incorporate the lessons that are being learned from dealing with the pandemic in the development of policy reforms and change management practices to protect the environment and the lives of their citizens.

References

Adams, J.G., and Walls, R.M. 2020. "Supporting the health care workforce during the COVID-19 global epidemic."*JAMA*, *323*(15): 1439–1440.https://doi.org/10.1001/jama.2020.3972.

Allan, B. B. 2017. "Second only to nuclear war: Science and the making of existential threat in global climate governance."*International Studies Quarterly, 61*(4) (December 20): 809–20.https://doi.org/10.1093/isq/sqx048.

Bénabou, R.,Falk, A., and Tirole, J. 2018. *Narratives, imperatives and moral reasoning*(working paper) (July). National Bureau of Economic Research.https://doi.org/10.3386/w24798.

Boin, R. 2005. "From Crisis to Disaster: Toward an Integrative Perspective." In *What Is a Disaster? New Answers to Old Questions,*edited by R. A. Perry and E. L. Quarantelli,155–172. Xlibris Press.

Fleming, N. 2020. "Coronavirus misinformation, and how scientists can help fight it."*Nature,* 583 (June 24): 155–156.https://doi.org/10.1038/d41586-020-01834-3.

Furst, S. A., and Cable, D. M. 2008. "Employee resistance to organizational change: managerial influence tactics and leader-member exchange."*Journal of Applied Psychology,* 93(2): 453–462. https://doi.org/10.1037/0021-9010.93.2.453.

Ford, J.D. & ford, L.W. (1995). The role of conversations in producing intentional change in orgnisations. *Academy of Management Review,* 20(3), 541-570.

Harvey, D. and Brown, D. R. 2001. *An Experimental Approach to Organization Development,* 6th ed. Prentice-Hall.

Kohll, A. 2020. "How one company is taking care of employees during COVID-19."*Forbes*.https://www.forbes.com/sites/alankohll/2020/04/06/how-one-company-is-taking-care-of-employees-during-covid-19/?sh=32bbf102488d.

Koliaki, C.,Tentolouris, A.,Eleftheriadou, I.,Melidonis, A.,Dimitriadis, G.,and Tentolouris, N. 2020. "Clinical management of Diabetes

Mellitus in the era of COVID-19: Practical issues, peculiarities and concerns."*Journal of Clinical Medicine,* 9(7): 2288.https://dx.doi.org/10.3390/jcm9072288.

Kotler, J. P. 1995. "Leading Change: Why transformation efforts fail." *HBR.* https://hbr.org/1995/05/leading-change-why-transformation-efforts-fail-2.

Lewin, K. 1951. *Field Theory in Social Science,* editedby D. Cartwright. Harper & Brothers.https://doi.org/10.1177%2F000271625127600135.

Lifton, R. 1983. *The Life of the Self: Toward a New Psychology.* Basic Books.

Miller, H. E. 2018. "Intuition and decision making in crisis situations."In *The Routledge Companion to Risk, Crisis and Security in Business,* 45–60. Taylor& Francis.https://doi.org/10.4324/9781315629520.

Oreg, S. 2003. "Resistance to change: Developing an individual differences measure."*Journal of Applied Psychology,* 88(4): 680–693.https://doi.org/10.1037/0021-9010.88.4.680.

Ram, I. G 2020. "Management philosophy: Toward an ethical worldview." In *Paradigm Shift in Management Philosophy: Future Challenges in Global Organizations,* edited B. S. Thakkar, 155–175. Palgrave Macmillan.

Ram, K. 2021. "A unified adaptive theory of global business culture." In *Culture in Global Businesses: Addressing National and Organizational Challe*nges, edited by B. S. Thakkar, 63–75. Palgrave Macmillan.

Rock, D. 2008. "SCARF: A brain-based model for collaborating with and Influencing Others."*NeuroLeadership Journal,* 1.http://dcntp.org/wp-content/uploads/2015/03/Readiness_for_change.pdf.

Ross, E. K. 1969. *On Death and Dying.* The Macmillan Company.

Simon, H. A. 1996. *The Sciences of the Artificial,* 3rd ed. MIT Press.

Sommer, P., Lukovic, E., Fagley, E., Long, D. R., Sobol, J. B., Heller, K., Moitra, V. K., Pauldine, R., O'Connor, M. F., Shahul, S., Nunnally, M. E., and Tung, A. 2020. Initial critical impressions of the critical care of COVID-19 patients in Seattle, New York City, and Chicago. *Anesthesia and Analgesia,* 131(1) (July): 55–60. https://doi.org/10.1213/ANE.0000000000004830.

Thorp, H. H. 2020. "Persuasive words are not enough."*Science, 368*(6498) (June 26): 1405.https://doi.org/10.1126/science.abd4085.

United Nations Development Programme. 2020. "COVID-19 and human development: Assessing the crisis, envisioning the recovery." http://hdr.undp.org/sites/default/files/covid-19_and_human_development_0.pdf.

Wen, T. 2020. "What makes people stop caring."*BBC News*(June 30). https://www.bbc.com/future/article/20200630-what-makes-people-stop-caring.

Wooten, L., and James, E. 2008. "Linking crisis management and leadership competencies: The role of human resource development."*Advances in Developing Human Resources* 10*(3)* (June 1): 352–379.https://doi.org/10.1177%2F1523422308316450.

CHAPTER 7

COVID-19: Clinician's Perspective and Impact on Healthcare Workers

by Akesh Thomas and Jay Mehta

Abstract

This chapter describes the experiences, struggles, and emotions of the doctors and nurses who helped the patients fight to survive COVID-19 during the pandemic. Healthcare workers (HCW) had to dive deep into their own emotions and professional ethics to deliver the best care.

The authors reviewed several scientific publications from reputable medical journals to compile the data. We analyzed clinical findings, treatment modality, and psychological reactions of the HCW. Our findings were fascinating. Doctors and nurses quickly learned the signs and symptoms of this new disease. COVID-19 is quite different from other viral illnesses. Critical care medicine (CCM) specialists also learned to differentiate the chest imaging, finding of COVID-19 pneumonia from bacterial pneumonia and other adult respiratory distress syndromes at a commendable pace.

Healthcare providers took the risk of their health. The work environment was stressful because scientific information was limited, and protective devices were in short supply. When these HCWs, particularly the females, went home, they had to take extra precautions to protect their family members, including children and aging parents. They also had the tragic experience of seeing their own colleagues getting sick.

While going through this crisis, they were shocked by the lack of education in the general public and their denial of the reality. Response from the political leaders and administration was equally frustrating. Unexpected clinical features like pulmonary embolism (PE) and cardiac involvement were new challenges. The healthcare professionals' attempt to keep up with evolving drug therapy and newer aspects of managing ventilators was quick and efficient. Changes in the healthcare system also affected the work environment and thus influenced the HCW, particularly those working in the ICU and ER.

In brief, this article is a review of the HCWs' experiences during the coronavirus pandemic. Lessons learned will help the HCW in the future and advance scientific knowledge about the clinical dilemma, psychological impact, and social burden that this pandemic posed to the practice of CCM. Lessons learned from this pandemic will improve our preparation for future epidemics of such magnitude.

Keywords: COVID-19, stress in ICU, doctors, and nurses in COVID-19, critical care medicine (CCM).

1.1 Introduction

Large-scale epidemics have influenced humanity throughout history. Communicable diseases became a leading cause of morbidity and mortality when the human race changed from hunter-gatherer to agrarian communities. Transmission of diseases like malaria, tuberculosis, smallpox, and influenza became easier when people started to live in clusters, forming towns and villages. About 5,000 years ago, a prehistoric village in China was wiped out by an epidemic. An archeologist named this site Hamin Mangha, meaning where a heap of burnt bones was found. The earliest recorded pandemic was perhaps in 430 BC. During the Peloponnesian war, the Spartans brought typhoid fever from Libya to the Athenian walls. Smallpox began with Huns, who infected Germans and Romans. Emperor Marcus Aurelius died from this illness. Black Death of AD 1350 that started in Asia spread to Europe, killing one-third of its population. Causative agent was Yersinia pestis. Doctors and nurses must have gone through a lot of psychological stress in those days though the documentation of such experiences is limited. In recent years, Spanish flu (1918) was responsible for 50 million deaths. Hong Kong flu of 1957 brought tragic death to some 1.1 million people. HIV/AIDS epidemic brought severe morbidity to more than 50 million human beings in the first ten years. While there is no vaccine, effective drug therapy has brought us a sigh of relief. Ebola and SARS have affected many in the last few years. With the novel coronavirus pandemic, we were caught with a sad surprise. Millions got sick, many millions have died, and the tragedy is not over yet. The impact of this horrible pandemic on HCWs and our healthcare system cannot be overlooked because it has posed some unique challenges.

2.0 Impact of COVID 19 on Healthcare System

On January 20, 2020, the first coronavirus case was reported in the United States in a man who returned from Wuhan, China. The first infection was reported in an HCW in the United States within the next week. Since then, more than 200,000 HCWs have been infected across the country in 2020 alone. In one study, the prevalence of positive SARS-CoV-2 test was 2,747 per 100,000, which was three-fold higher than in the general population (1). In hospitals where the personal protective equipment (PPE) supply was inadequate, the infection rate was higher. Minorities were at a fivefold risk of infection compared to the general population. This data is likely an underestimate of the real numbers considering the significant gaps in reporting and data collection. This has affected the life of HCWs in all aspects. The previous experience of the Ebola outbreak probably helped both the scientists and clinicians; however, posttraumatic stress disorder and other mental health problems among health care professionals remained an under-recognized fact during the Ebola, SARS, and COVID pandemic (Hong et al. 2009).

2.1 COVID-19 Risk

In 2019, 18.6 million people were working in the healthcare industry at different levels of exposure to the virus. The Center for Disease Control (CDC) reported 200,000 cases and 790 deaths among the HCP by mid-November 2020. Most likely, this is an underestimate because the healthcare status of only 25% of the HCP was known at the time of this report. More than half (53%) of confirmed cases were among HCP of color (26% Black, 12% Hispanic, and 9% Asian). Nurses and those in direct contact with the patient were at the highest risk of getting infected; some of them had limited access to PPE. Black

HCP and their family adults were less likely to accept vaccination compared to the white HCP and their family members (Hamel et al. 2021).

A report from Southern Iran (Fars's province) showed that out of 4854 PCR testes for COVID-19, 273 of HCW (5.62%) had a positive result, which was more than double, as reported in the general population (Shoja et al. 2020). Nurses had a much higher risk than other HCW. Despite using the masks and following the safety protocol, the HCWs were at a very high risk of getting infected; thus, the fear of HCW is quite understandable.

Stress level: From the very beginning of the pandemic, HCWs were at a high level of mental stress. Rapid spread, along with the largely unknown nature of the disease and absence of curative treatment, added to the stress. In addition to the limited availability of PPE, shortage of trained medical staff, fatigue, and fear, the critical care specialists had the difficult task of keeping up with changing recommendations for the treatment of COVID-19. Dexamethasone and Remdesivir were used as the immunosuppressant based on limited scientific data. The use of hydroxychloroquine was controversial from the very beginning, but the patients and their family members frequently demanded this drug. New mechanical ventilation techniques for respiratory failure were evolving when the patients were hypoxic and seriously ill. Artificial ventilation in the prone position was started based on the logic that redistribution of blood flow will improve oxygenation; however, the scientific proof was lacking, and treating ill patients when clinical signs, symptoms, and specific treatment were almost unknown increased mental stress. Although many cities had initiated lockdowns and travel restrictions to reduce the spread of infection, HCWs were obviously still expected to continue to provide service. The lack of enough PPE added to the stress among HCWs at this time. Scholars from all around the world called for a better understanding of the psychosocial problems caused by the pandemic (Duan and Zhu 2020; Holmes et al. 2020).

The most common psychiatric disorders diagnosed among HCWs in a review by Cabarkapa et al. were posttraumatic stress syndrome, depression, and anxiety (Cabarkapa et al. 2020). Somatization was another psychiatric condition identified among HCWs during the pandemic (Xiaoming et al. 2020); in fact, one study found nearly half of the HCWs having some form of somatic complaint (Hong et al. 2020). HCWs' burnout was another significant issue that was unaccounted for in some of these studies.

At the individual level, healthcare providers had adverse psychological effects identified in multiple areas, including anxiety, depression, and stress (Dong et al. 2021; Ni et al. 2020). The physical stress from the increase in working hours added to the mental stress (Cao et al. 2020). Posttraumatic stress disorder has become more pronounced among HCW later in the pandemic. Unfortunately, it is expected to continue to impact the lives of many HCWs.

Lack of sleep was another important concern among HCWs. It was caused by the physical stress from increased working hours and lack of adequate rest caused by work-related chronic anxiety. The lack of sleep was so common and had so much impact that a new term was coined, COVID insomnia. Although all these mental stress-related symptoms were noticed in various community members, the problems were more prevalent and severe among the HCW. Many doctors and nurses largely quarantined themselves from their family and friends during the pandemic, adding to a significant lack of social support and mental stress. While many citizens throughout the USA live with fear and uncertainty, many workers could work from their homes. Essential workers, including HCW who could not work from home, must risk exposure to the virus every day. Healthcare workers in ICUs experienced a work environment that has been compared to a war zone where they witness the tragedy and risk their own lives. Mental Health America (MHA)conducted a survey from June to September 2020 to understand the mental health risk of the HCW. They received 1,119 responses. Here are the findings: 93% of HCW were experiencing stress. Seventy-seven percent reported frustration. seventy-six percent of HCW with children reported their worries about exposing their children when they go home after an exhausting day.

Female HCWs were at particular risk of mental stress during the pandemic. Most studies found that female healthcare workers had significantly increased psychiatric complications attributed to the pandemic (Pouralizadeh et al. 2020; Romero et al. 2020). Separation from young children and family may have been a significant factor, especially since the vast majority of the study's population were nurses; female HCWs significantly outnumber male HCWs in nursing jobs throughout the world. Suicidal ideation was also found more among female HCWs during the COVID-19 pandemic (Xiaoming et al. 2021).

The COVID-19 pandemic had a significant impact on the family dynamics. The parent-child relationship is the most affected part of the family during the pandemic. Parental mental health and stress, lack of time investment from parents, changes in the way parent-child time was spent, and reduced quality of parent-child interactions are all factored in. This was particularly true for small families and those with poor financial support. Families of many HCWs had to make arrangements for childcare after schools were closed. Many HCWs had difficulty in explaining their distancing from family to their children. Among the HCWs we have interviewed, we saw various shades of anxiety, frustration, and sleep deprivation. While most were dedicated and did their duty with due diligence, few decided to take early retirement or take leave of absence, augmenting the shortage of skilled workers.

The financial implications of the COVID-19 pandemic were different across the spectrum for HCWs and healthcare systems. While the majority had a financial crisis, a few gained financial benefit during the pandemic. A survey by the Duke University Clinical Research Institute in February 2021 reported 34 % of HCWs were worried about meeting financial obligations while about 9% reported furlough or forced leave of absence (Duke Clinical Research Group 2021).

The change in childcare costs and the rising cost of housing escalated the financial crisis for HCWs. When elective procedures and nonemergency treatments were stopped by hospitals, there were many physicians and nurses who were forced to do an emergency room or critical care shifts after being in practice at a different specialty for years. The hospitals were also at a significant loss since the lion's share of hospitals earnings comes from elective surgical or medical procedures rather than emergency and critical care. The American hospital association had estimated a financial impact of about 202.6 billion revenue loss during the time of the pandemic (Kaye et al. 2020).

COVID-19's impact on different races was drastically different. While in the general population, blacks suffered more death from COIVD-19 (Chowkwanyun and Reed 2020), the disparities in the healthcare sector were no different. In our experience, the hospital workers who were furloughed or lost their job were primarily racial minorities; this can be partly due to the greater number of blacks and other minorities working in housekeeping services, food preparation and serving, and transportation and moving. A study by Rogers et al. found that black workers had an increased risk of infection by the COVID virus essentially due to the nature of their jobs (Rogers et al.

2020). The psychological and financial impact was also more on racial and ethnic minorities during the pandemic.

3.0 HCW in Long-Term Care Facility

In the early phase of the pandemic, high morbidity and mortality were noticed among the residents of nursing homes and skilled care facilities. Many of these patients were elderly and had comorbidity. Some of them were immunocompromised. Employees working in such facilities were also at a high risk of getting the infection. In early August, 671,237 residents were reported to have confirmed COVID-19 infection, leading to 134,071 deaths. CDC report during the same time indicated that 608,606 staff members working at various long-term care facilities had positive COVID-19 test with 1,880 deaths. There was a shortage of isolation facilities, negative pressure rooms, and various protective devices for the nurses, respiratory therapists, and other staff members. In the later phase, the infection rate declined as the preventive measures were in force and vaccines became available.

3.1 Impact on Healthcare System

COIVD-19 affected different healthcare systems in different ways. While most primary care clinics had to close at least at the beginning of the pandemic, many urgent care centers had an increase in the number of patients, and the hospitals had a mixed impact based on the service. The American board of family physicians had projected about 15 billion revenue loss for primary care practices. The situation improved slightly after Medicaid and Medicare lifted the restrictions on reimbursement of telehealth visits. But it took time for most primary care practices to arrange the setup needed and training for a telehealth visit; some clinics never achieved this. There was also a considerable variation in the adaptation of telehealth practices based on the location. Senior citizens, especially in rural areas, were slow to adapt to the telehealth visits, so did practitioners. All insurances were not covering phone calls as telehealth visits which added to the problem. The federal government's CARES Act was cited by many primary care practice owners as something which sustained their practice during the crisis. Access to PPE was not easy for primary care practices while many large hospitals managed to arrange the PPE they needed.

When hospitals and clinics faced the acute crisis after the initial standstill, hospital management and clinicians adopted different methods and techniques to tackle the situation. N95 mask was not known to many patients outside the research and healthcare sector before the pandemic; this has become a household name by the end of last year. The initial change for the healthcare sectors was to find adequate PPE for HCWs. Hospitals promptly redirected the PPE kits, gloves, and protective gowns from elective surgical supplies and clinics to COVID treating wards. The lack of adequate N95 masks prompted hospitals to urge HCWs to use one N95 for a period of twenty-four hours or more for multiple patients. To the extreme, some hospitals came up with a system to sterilize the N95 mask using ultraviolet rays, and surprisingly, this did not reduce the performance of N95 masks (Zhao et al. 2020).

A shortage of regular surgical and procedural masks for healthcare professional use had also existed at the beginning of the pandemic when the public bought in masks (Ji et al. 2020). Shortage of adequate beds for COVID-19 infected patients forced hospitals to close other units and convert them to isolation/COVID-19 units; this was not enough in areas like the Northeastern United States at the beginning of the pandemic where temporary tents were made outside of hospitals to treat COVID-19 patients. The US Navy had to deploy its hospital ships to the Northeastern

United States at the peak of the pandemic. Mechanical ventilation support was the only treatment option for coronavirus-infected patients initially, but the supply of mechanical ventilators in the country was not enough. The federal government moved mechanical ventilators out from its stockpile to states in need. Similarly, states with less infection rate lend their ventilators to states with high infection rate, but none of these efforts solved the inadequate supply of ventilators in the beginning. Hospitals adopted newer techniques of using more high-flow nasal cannula (an oxygen supply through the nasal cannula with a very high oxygen flow rate compared to regular nasal cannula) and experts in medical research invented the technology to split one ventilator between two patients.

COVID-19 also had a significant impact on medical education and training just like or more than any other education during the pandemic. Medical students were asked to stay out of the hospital for a while. When PPE was in short supply, medical students had to give way to personals who were directly involved in the treatment of the patients. Many institutions stopped taking students from other medical schools for elective rotations, which was a major source of knowledge sharing and networking opportunity for medical students from schools with less advanced facilities. Reduced number of medical students on the service increased the work of residents in training and worsened their sense of isolation. The closing of elective procedures and nonessential services also affected the quality of medical education during this pandemic. Similarly, residents and fellows who are supposedly be seeing a wide variety of pathology during their training period were essentially limited to more and more coronavirus cases during the pandemic. The ancillary medical education courses, including nursing, physical therapy, occupational therapy, speech therapy, optometry, operating room technician, etc., were all affected by the coronavirus pandemic.

Many training programs experienced a substantial delay in starting their training for the 2021 academic year.

Resources and funding were redirected to virology research, especially COVID-related research, which was essential at the time (Harper et al. 2020). This has created a break in research in many other areas, including cancer research. On the brighter side, scientific advancements like the mRNA vaccine took a leap and provided a great benefit to humanity at large. Many countries, including the United States, have realized the need for better preventive measures. The importance of primary care physicians was reinforced once again. The need for a strong public health system became obvious as the pandemic advanced in higher morbidity and mortality.

The COVID-19 pandemic affected the functioning of some essential but noninfectious disease medical specialties with devastating consequences to the patients. Most noteworthy is the near-complete shutdown of cancer care in many places at the beginning. Cancer patients, especially after radiation or chemotherapy, are at increased risk of infection; this created concern among patients and providers alike, and they avoided hospitals more than most other kinds of patients until alternate arrangements were made by hospitals. Similarly, new diagnosis and initiation of treatment were also delayed significantly across the nation (Patt et al. 2020).

Maternal and child healthcare was another area of healthcare affected significantly by the COVID-19 pandemic (Akseer et al. 2020); pregnancy and labor for the mother and neonatal period for the newborn are crucial periods, which require constant healthcare services support and education. Similarly, other areas like hospice and palliative care services, mental health services, etc., were also affected by the pandemic.

Social and psychological support should be provided to the HCWs more than normal during pandemics like COIVD-19 (Ni et al. 2020). Active mind-body therapies like yoga, tai chi, were found to have a positive impact on mental health, especially posttraumatic stress disorder. These are low-cost methods that can be implemented even during a crisis like the COVID-19 pandemic. The available data is mostly on the immediate effects of the COVID-19 pandemic, but many of the psychological impacts on HCWs may have a prolonged course. More longitudinal studies and follow-ups are needed to assess the complete effect.

Once peak COVID-19 infections settled down, healthcare systems must address problems such as the overstock of mechanical ventilators, the fate of workers who were furloughed, excess personal protection equipment, HCWs who refuse to get vaccinated, mask mandate in the hospital, and a host of other issues that are the result of the measures taken during the onset and escalation of the pandemic.

3.2 The Third Wave of the Pandemic

The greatest infection surges and COVID-19 related deaths had passed by mid-2021, yet surges of COVID-19 variants, such as delta and omicron continued to raise concerns as to when the pandemic would end. Viruses go through mutations frequently, but this delta variant has certain unique features that have created new problems and the omicron variant emerged with less mortality yet with higher infection rates and different symptoms. The COIVD-19 treatment units and COVID-19-only intensive care units, which were thought closed forever, have reopened in response to the emergence of variants and mental stress and frustration continue to affect HCWs.

The delta (B.1.617.2) variant is a genetically mutated coronavirus that was first identified in India at the end of 2020 and has rapidly spread across the globe. The delta variant is believed to be at least twice potent in infection rate compared to the initial coronavirus. Although the vaccine effectiveness is believed to be almost the same as that of against initial (alpha) coronavirus variant (Bernal et al. 2021), the speed of infection and more symptomatic disease is making the situation catastrophic. According to the CDC, more than 90% of the new cases in July and August 2021 are from the delta variant. Delta variant is more infectious, and the mean age of those admitted to the hospital is lower than what we experienced in the early months of 2021. Vaccine efficacy seems to be declining from 91% to 66%. Scientists are not clear if the mutant variant is responsible for the increase in cases among vaccinated people. Those who received the vaccine in the early part of its availability might experience the declining efficacy of the vaccine because of the declining antibody level. During this third wave of the pandemic, unvaccinated were 29 times more likely to be hospitalized than vaccinated individuals. A letter to the *New England Journal of Medicine* published on August 18, 2021, reported breakthrough infections of BNT 162b2 (Pfizer-Bio-N-tech) and mRNA-1273 (Moderna) vaccinated hospital employees in Germany (Lange et al. 2021). Out of 1,137 vaccinated HCW, four immuno-competent women (0.35%) had a breakthrough infection. Most of them developed the infection and the symptoms in the late duration after the second dose of the vaccine (average 62 days), and the viral shedding continued for 32 days as tested by the gene testing. This infection rate was higher than that reported in the phase three trial (0.05%). As the schools open in August, the school systems are facing new problems, where some parents want mask mandate and others oppose it. Pediatric hospitals throughout the country are experiencing a surge in the admission rate. A New Orleans children's hospital had so many new COVID-19 cases that a federal *surge team* was called in to help the exhausted staff. In another hospital in TN (hospital: A), the administration raises the nurse's salaries to retain them. This created discontent among Respiratory therapists (RT). A nearby hospital (hospital-B) offered an incentive payment to the new RTs recruited, resulting in an acute shortage of RT in hospital A. This third wave of COVID-19 is posing many new challenges with no sight of light at the end of the tunnel.

COVID-19 vaccine: Unlike the influenza vaccine, the COVID-19 vaccine is an mRNA-based vaccine. It is an extraordinary achievement that the scientists were able to develop this vaccine in a short time.

In March 2021, the Houston Methodist hospital mandated COVID-19 vaccination for all its employees, the first of its kind mandate in the country; after a brief legal battle, the hospital held its position. Indiana University was the following major organization that made the COVID-19 vaccine mandatory, and that was followed by the veteran's admiration hospitals mandating COVID-19 employers although the controversy around this may continue for a while.

4.0 A Few Case Studies throughout the Pandemic Period (The locations were changed to protect patient privacy)

4.3 Case Study 1:

A woman graduated from nursing school in 2018 and since then has been working as an intensive care unit nurse in a large hospital system in New Jersey. She is a single mother of two young boys, 3 and 5. When she heard about the new virus infection in China and Washington, she did not expect it to reach New Jersey too soon. Earlier in 2020, after the first coronavirus cases were reported in her hospital, she was horrified, and she describes it as the moment where her life stood still. She was constantly afraid to go back to her kids after working in the hospital more than her own health in the face of the unknown virus infection. Later, when the job stress escalated, she had to ask her mother to help with her children at home. Although in her late sixties, her mother came to her house to help her. She still questions her decision to call her mother from a non-reported coronavirus suburb of Kentucky to the then center of coronavirus infection in the Northeastern United States, but she had no other options. The story of the coronavirus pandemic is also the story of thousands of nurses and other HCWs like her. It changed the healthcare system and life of HCWs as never before.

Discussion:

Epidemics and pandemics can have varying effects on the life of different people. It influences physical and mental health, financial, social, and even cultural aspects of an individual and society. HCWs and low socioeconomic status groups are the two most vulnerable groups adversely affected by this pandemic. In this article, we will explore certain aspects of the coronavirus pandemic and its impact on HCWs and hospitals, especially in the United States.

Case Study 2: March 2020

An 86-year-old man moved to a nursing home nearby the small town in Massachusetts, where he lived for almost all his life after a recent fall breaking his hip bone. The nursing home stay was expected to be for a few months until his son could take care of him, and he was improving rapidly than expected. He developed a low-grade fever and minimal cough early in March 2020, which progressed to severe shortness of breath in three days. He was taken to the nearby hospital emergency room where his oxygen saturation was found to be in the sixties (normally, it should be in the high nineties). The emergency room physician obtained a chest X-ray (image 4) that showed haziness throughout his lung fields. He tested positive for the COVID virus; he was put on a ventilator for about a week, and later his condition worsened and he passed away, never reaching his home. Following that, an outbreak of COVID virus infection was reported in the nursing home, killing several of its residents.

Discussion:

This case illustrates the tragedy in the long-term care facility. The infection rate was high, and the elderly were at a high risk of developing serious pneumonia. The mortality rate was high in the early stage of the pandemic mainly because the elderly patients are at a high risk of developing pneumonia and respiratory failure leading to death. Isolation facility was limited in most nursing homes; hence, the transmission could not be prevented. HCW were faced with the additional risk of infection, and their work environment was very stressful.

Case Study 3: July 2021

A 32-year-old carpenter from a small city in Alabama and his family were very skeptical of the COVID-19 vaccine and decided to wait a year before taking the vaccine. He was happy that he never got the infection and went out with his work and daily life as before COVID after the regulations were lifted by the state authority. Late in July 2021, he started to have a mild cough and tiredness; he went and saw his primary care physician, and he tested positive for COVID-19 infection.

He went home and did fine for three days until he became unconscious, and his wife had to call 911 to take him to the hospital. While he arrived in the hospital, his blood oxygen saturation levels were in the forties. He was placed on a mechanical ventilator initially and then was transferred to a higher center for extracorporeal membrane oxygenation. After about a month, he was able to go home, but he suffered from a severe neurological deficit now, unable to communicate or recognize anyone, including his family.

Discussion:

This case report demonstrates the serious challenge that the patient, family members, and the HCW had to face in such patients who develop complications of COVID infection. The cardiac or neurological complication of this disease poses a long-term care issue in patients who get better from the pulmonary illness from the COVID. Doctors and nurses felt helpless when patients developed such complications in spite of the best care that they tried to deliver. This case also illustrates the rapid change in the clinical status that some patients go through, thus creating the unexpected risk in the management of such cases.

Case Study 4: July 2021

A 56-year-old radio talk show host presented to the ER with a cough and fever of one-week duration. In the month of May and June, he had discouraged people from using masks, vaccination, and various preventive practices recommended by the CDC. He did not get vaccinated even though it was easily available in the health department only a few miles from the place of his work. His symptoms deteriorated to dyspnea and low oxygen saturation. He required admission to the hospital. In a few short hours, his condition worsened, and he was transferred to the

ICU. Despite several days of treatment on the ventilator and treatment like corticosteroid, immunosuppressive drugs, and ventilator support, his CT chest showed worsening of Covid pneumonia. He required ventilation in the prone position. When pneumonia is in the posterior part of the lung, changing the position of the patient improves the blood circulation to the healthy part of the lung, which is the anterior part of the upper and lower lobes. He and his family now had a new perspective on vaccination and the use of masks, but the patient could not talk to educate the public. He regretted the misguidance that he had promoted. Unfortunately, his realization was too late. When the traditional ventilator therapy failed to improve his oxygenation and his medical condition deteriorated, the family requested an ECMO ventilator, a special treatment that was not available in the county hospital. His medical condition was so delicate that he could not be transferred to a tertiary care hospital. Even if he became stable, the nearby tertiary hospital did not have advanced ECMO machines available to treat this patient. After a few days of continued treatment, he expired.

Discussion:

This case presents a story of a patient who had misguided many and ignored the public health recommendations. He did not use a mask or vaccination to protect himself. In the end, he came to regret his actions. This situation created unique emotions in the minds of the doctors and nurses who took care of him. He had the opportunity to educate the public and encourage them to use masks and social distancing, thus reducing the number of active cases in this region.

Secondly, his medical condition deteriorated rapidly despite excellent medical care; it was too late to transfer him to a tertiary care facility. Such experiences add to the mental agony of the patients, family members, and HCW. This case emphasizes crisis management and stresses that the hospital-based doctors and nurses experience daily as they take care of patients in such difficult situations.

This and several such cases with tragic ends have created frustration in the mind and the heart of the clinicians working in ICU and critical care medicine. It is a difficult task to take care of patients with respiratory failure from Covid pneumonia when the scientific knowledge of this clinical illness and effective treatment is rapidly changing. Nurses and doctors have faced many such challenges and worked in an environment that poses additional risks to their own physical and mental health.

5.0 Concluding Remarks

COVID-19 has posed a great challenge to the healthcare system in general and the medical profession in particular. Medical professionalism is changing with an ever-increasing gap between traditional teaching and the realities of modern medical practice. This pandemic has forced substantial demands on the already understaffed and overstretched healthcare system. Practice safety has led to an increase in the use of PPE devices. Mask, frequent handwashing, and social distancing have become a new normal in almost all the hospitals and clinics across the USA. Liability issues have taken a new meaning. Pre-visit patient screening is almost universal in all the clinics, ER, and doctor's offices. Regular disinfecting surfaces during and after seeing each patient visit is practiced daily. To minimize the direct contact hours, telehealth has become a new specialty. Physicians spend a lot more time in front of the laptop to check the reports and contact their patients through email, tax, or patient portals. Patients who are not sick enough to be admitted are monitored by telemedicine, which is used not only by certified doctors but by nurses, nurse clinicians, and physician assistants. There is *technology fatigue* in the eyes of many doctors and nurses. Patient flow has become very important. Hospitals have become quite aware of the need to address physician well-being, an important resource for today and tomorrow. Doctors, nurses, and support staff are vital resources for the future if the quality of healthcare has to be maintained in the coming years. Many changes are in place to minimize the transmission of infection in the healthcare setting, at the same time controlling the waste and maintaining efficiency. Future research will be essential to answering questions like are these changes effective, how do we maintain the quality of care while adopting these changes? A well-planned research, continued vigilance, and a strong commitment to high-quality, cost-effective patient care are our best hope as we learn from this costly and disastrous pandemic.

References

Akseer, N., Kandru, G., Keats, E. C., and Bhutta, Z. A. 2020. "COVID-19 pandemic and mitigation strategies: Implications for maternal and child health and nutrition." *The American Journal of Clinical Nutrition, 112* (2) (June 19): 251–256. https://doi.org/10.1093/ajcn/nqaa171.

Bernal, J. L., Andrews, N., Gower, C., Gallagher, E., Simmons, R., Thelwall, S., Stowe, J., Tessier, E., Groves, N., Dabrera, G., Myers, R., Campbell, C. N. J., Amirthalingam, G., Edmunds, M., Zambon, M., Brown, K. E., Hopkins, S., Chand, M., and Ramsay, M. 2021. "Effectiveness of COVID-19 vaccines against the B.1.617.2 (Delta) variant." *New England Journal of Medicine*, 385 (7) (August 12): 585–594. https://doi.org/10.1056/NEJMoa2108891.

Cabarkapa, S., Nadjidai, S. E., Murgier, J., Ng, C. H. 2020. The psychological impact of COVID-19 and other viral epidemics on frontline healthcare workers and ways to address it: A rapid systematic review. *Brain, Behavior, and Immunity—Health,* 8 (October). https://doi.org/10.1016/j.bbih.2020.100144.

Cao, J., Wei, J., Zhu, H., Duan, Y., Geng, W., Hong, X., Jiang, J., Zhao, X., and Zhu, B. 2020. "A study of basic needs and psychological wellbeing of medical workers in the fever clinic of a tertiary general hospital in Beijing during the COVID-19 outbreak." *Psychotherapy and Psychosomatics,* 89 (4) (July): 252–254. https://doi.org/10.1159/000507453.

Chowkwanyun, M., and Reed, A. 2020. "Racial health disparities and COVID-19—Caution and context." *New England Journal of Medicine,* 383 (3): 201–203. https://doi.org/10.1056/nejmp2012910.

Dong, F., Liu, H. L., Yang, M., Lu, C., Dai, N., Zhang, Y., Robinson, N., and Liu, J. 2021. "Immediate psychosocial impact on healthcare workers during COVID-19 pandemic in China: A systematic review and meta-analysis." *Frontiers in Psychology* (May 28). https://doi.org/10.3389/fpsyg.2021.645460.

Duan, L., and Zhu, G. 2020. Psychological interventions for people affected by the COVID-19 epidemic. *Lancet Psychiatry,* 7 (4) (April 7):300–302. https://doi.org/10.1016/S2215-0366(20)30073-0.

Duke Clinical Research Group. 2021. "The hidden cost of COVID-19 impact on healthcare heroes' finances." *CISION PR Newswire* (February 11). https://www.prnewswire.com/news-releases/the-hidden-cost-of-covid-19-impact-on-healthcare-heroes-finances-301226472.html.

Hamel, L., Lopes, L., Kearney, A., Kirzinger, A., Sparks, G., Stokes, M., and Brodie, M. 2021. *KFF COVID-19 Vaccine Monitor: Parents and the Pandemic* (August 11). https://www.kff.org/coronavirus-covid-19/poll-finding/kff-covid-19-vaccine-monitor-parents-and-the-pandemic/.

Harper, L., Kalfa, N., Beckers, G. M. A., Kaefer, M., Nieuwhof-Leppink, A., J., Fossum, M., Herbst, K. W., and Bagli, D. 2020. "The impact of COVID-19 on research." *Journal of Pediatric Urology,* 16 (5): 715–716. https://doi.org/10.1016/j.jpurol.2020.07.002.

Holmes, E. A., O'Connor, R. C., Perry, V. H., Tracey, I., Wessely, S., Arseneault, L., Ballard, C., Christensen, H., Silver, R. C., Everall, I., Ford, T., John, A., Kabir, T, King, K., Madan, I., Michie, S., Przybylski, A. K., Shafran, R., Sweeney, A., . . . Bullmore, E. 2020. "Multidisciplinary research priorities for the COVID-19 pandemic: A call for action for mental health science." *Lancet Psychiatry,* 7 (6) (June 1):547–560. https://doi.org/10.1016/S2215-0366(20)30168-1.

Hong, S., Ai, M., Xu, X., Wang, W., Chen, J., Zhang, Q., Wang, L., Kuang, L. 2021. Immediate psychological impact on nurses working at 42 government-designated hospitals during COVID-19 outbreak in China: A cross-sectional study. *Nursing Outlook,* 69 (1) (January 1), 6–12. https://doi.org/10.1016/j.outlook.2020.07.007.

Hong, X., Currier, G. W., Zhao, X., Jiang, Y., Zhou, W., and Wei, J. 2009. "Posttraumatic stress disorder in convalescent severe acute respiratory syndrome patients: A 4-year follow-up study." *General Hospital Psychiatry,* 31 (6) (November-December): 546–554. https://doi.org/10.1016/j.genhosppsych.2009.06.008.

Ji, D., Fan, L., Li, X., and Ramakrishna, S. 2020. "Addressing the worldwide shortages of face masks." *BMC Materials,* 2 (9). https://doi.org/10.1186/s42833-020-00015-w.

Kaye, A. D., Okeagu, C. N., Pham, A. D., Silva, R. A., Hurley, J. J., Arron, B. L., Sarfraz, N., Lee, H. N., Ghali, G. E., Gamble, J. W., Liu, H., Urman, R. D., and Cornett, E. M. 2021. "Economic impact of COVID-19 pandemic on healthcare facilities and systems: International perspectives." *Best Practice & Research Clinical Anaesthesiology,* 35 (3): 293–306. https://doi.org/10.1016/j.bpa.2020.11.009.

Lange, B., Gerigk, M., and Tenenbaum, T. 2021. "Breakthrough Infections in BNT162b2-vaccinated health care workers." *New England Journal of Medicine*, 385, 1145–1146. https://www.nejm.org/doi/10.1056/NEJMc2108076.

Nguyen, L. H., Drew, D. A., Graham, M. S., Joshi, A. D., Guo, C., Ma, W., Mehta, R. S., Warner, E. T., Sikavi, D. R., Lo, C., Kwon, S., Song, M., Mucci, L. A., Stampfer, M. J., Willett, W. C., Eliassen, A. H., Hart, J. E., Chavarro, J. E., Rich-Edwards, J. W., . . . Chan, A. T. 2020. "Risk of COVID-19 among front-line health-care workers and the general community: A prospective cohort study." *The Lancet Public Health,* 5 (9) (September 1). https://doi.org/10.1016/s2468-2667(20)30164-x.

Ni, M. Y., Yang, L., Leung, C. M. C., Li, N., Yao, X. I., Wang, Y., Leung, G. M., Cowling, B.J., and Liao, Q. 2020. Mental health, risk factors, and social media use during the COVID-19 epidemic and Cordon Sanitaire among the community and health professionals in Wuhan, China: Cross-sectional survey. *Journal of Medical Internet Research Mental Health,* 7 (5) (May 12). https:/doi.org/10.2196/19009.

Patt, D., Gordan, L., Diaz, M., Okon, T., Grady, L., Harmison, M., Markward, N., Sullivan, M., Peng, J., and Zhou, A. 2020. "Impact of COVID-19 on cancer care: How the pandemic is delaying cancer diagnosis and treatment for American seniors." *JCO Clinical Cancer Informatics,* 4, 1059–1071. https://doi.org/10.1200/CCI.20.00134.

Pouralizadeh, M., Bostani, Z., Maroufizadeh, S., Ghanbari, A., Khoshbakht, M., Alavi, S. A., and Ashrafi, S. 2020. "Anxiety and depression and the related factors in nurses of Guilan university of medical sciences hospitals during COVID-19: A web-based cross-sectional study." *International Journal of Africa Nursing Sciences,* 13, 1–6. https://doi.org/10.1016/j.ijans.2020.100233.

Rogers, T., Rogers, C., VanSant-Webb, E., Gu, L., Yan, B., and Qeadan, F. 2020. "Racial disparities in COVID-19 mortality among essential workers in the United States." *World Medical and Health Policy,* 12 (3) (August 5): 311–327. https://doi.org/10.1002/wmh3.358.

Romero, C., Delgado, C., Catalá, J., Ferrer, C., Errando, C., Iftimi, A, Benito, A., de Andrés, J., Otero, M., and the PSIMCOV group. 2020. "COVID-19 psychological impact in 3109 healthcare workers in Spain: the PSIMCOV group." *Psychological Medicine,* (May 14) 1–7. https://doi.org/10.1017/S0033291720001671

Shoja, E., Aghamohammadi, V., Bazyar, H., Moghaddam, h. R., Nasiri, K., Dashti, M., Choupani, A., Garaee, M., Aliasgharzadeh, S., and Asgari, A. 2020. "COVID-19 effects on the workload of Iranian healthcare workers." *BMC Public Health,* 20, 1636. https://doi.org/10.1186/s12889-020-09743-w.

Xiaoming, X., Ming, A., Su, H., Wo, W., Jianmei, C., Qi, Z., Hua, H., Xuemei, L., Lixia, W., Jun, C., Lei, S., Zhen, L., Lian, D.,

Jing, L., Handan, Y., Haitang, Q., Xiaoting, H., Xiaorong, C., Ran, . . . Li, K. 2020. "The psychological status of 8817 hospital workers during COVID-19 Epidemic: A cross-sectional study in Chongqing." *Journal of Affective Disorders, 276* (November 1): 555–561. https://doi.org/10.1016/j.jad.2020.07.092.

Zhao, Z., Zhang, Z., Lanzarini-Lopes, M., Sinha, S., Rho, H., Herckes, P., and Westerhoff, P. 2020. "Germicidal ultraviolet light does not damage or impede performance of N95 masks upon multiple uses." *Environmental Science and Technology Letters, 7* (8) (June 24): 600–605. https://doi.org/10.1021/acs.estlett.0c00416.

CHAPTER 8

Understanding the Effects of Coronavirus from a Virological and Public Health Perspective

by Kunj R. Patel

Abstract

Understanding the virology of the COVID-19 virus is paramount to recognizing its potency, transmission vectors, diagnosis, and prognosis. Such an understanding will help reduce misinformation regarding the virus. This chapter aims to sequentially describe the responses from the medical community to the coronavirus since discovering its origin in Wuhan, China, in November 2019. It also aims to describe the biology of the predecessors of COVID-19 (severe acute respiratory syndrome and Middle East respiratory syndrome) and how these iterations of the virus incorporate themselves into human and animal cells. Furthermore, this chapter explains how medical professionals test for the virus and a genomic explanation of how the results of the test are interpreted. This chapter also analyzes the genomics of vaccine development of COVID-19 and how this process differs from the nine traditional forms of virus vaccine development. In addition, the mechanisms of action of eight different vaccines (some of them are still undergoing clinical trials) are analyzed in this chapter. Lastly, this chapter provides a public health perspective to earlier coronavirus outbreaks in China (severe acute respiratory syndrome) and the Middle East (Middle East respiratory syndrome). It will also project how successful policies to curtail the effects of those epidemics can be applied to a pandemic situation to provide the greatest benefit to the most people. Providing a technical background of how the medical community is combating the virus since its discovery in 2019. Explaining how the virus works can inform people and allow them to analyze which measures should be taken to combat the COVID-19 pandemic. In addition, providing public awareness can also inform people on how to best prepare themselves for the rise of future disease outbreaks since microorganisms and viruses are known to evolve faster than medical scientists can develop methods of treatment.

Keywords: COVID-19, vaccine, PCR (polymerase chain reaction), coronavirus, SARS (severe acute respiratory syndrome), MERS (Middle East respiratory syndrome)

1.0 Introduction

COVID-19 is part of a greater viral category of coronaviruses. It is a positive-strand RNA virus, meaning that it does not require a reverse transcriptase enzyme to replicate itself. Instead, it can make a complementary RNA copy quickly. Coronaviruses are distinguished by their crown-like arrangement of their surface proteins when observed by an electron microscope, hence the prefix corona. Symptoms of all coronaviruses are generally related to the respiratory tract of humans, such as shortness of breath and pneumonia-like symptoms. Other notable viruses in this category include SARS (severe acute respiratory syndrome) and MERS (Middle East respiratory syndrome). As of August 2021, there are seven types of coronaviruses that have been known to infect humans (229E, NL63, OC43, HKU1, MERS-CoV, SARS-CoV, and SARS-CoV-2). The most common coronavirus infections in humans are 229E, NL63, OC43, and HKU1. All human coronaviruses have been found to be types of alpha-coronaviruses or beta-coronaviruses. COVID-19 was found to be a beta-coronavirus. In epidemiological studies of alpha coronaviruses, symptoms of coronavirus were found to be milder than that of SARS or MERS. According to the NIH, the receptor-binding domains of beta coronaviruses are different from alpha coronaviruses. In other words, beta coronaviruses have a different spike protein structure than alpha coronaviruses.

1.1 rigins of COVID-19

On December 31, 2019, the Wuhan Municipal Health Commission in China reported 27 pneumonia cases clustered with findings of fever, breathing difficulties, and chest X-ray infiltrations. Since the etiology (the causes or set of causes) of the virus was not yet known, these cases were merely reported as pneumonia cases. According to structural analyses of the virus, the genome of COVID-19 most strongly resembled another virus named BatCoVRaTG13 (96.3% match) commonly found in bats, which is a clear indication that the virus likely came from an infected bat. However, the probability of the virus transferring directly from bat to human is very unlikely according to structural analyses of the virus. In fact, based on the analysis of the glycoproteins that are found on the surface in the capsid, a protein cage of the virus, snakes were concluded to be the most likely intermediary transmission vector from bats to humans.

1.2 Public Health

Infectivity is the ability of a virus to begin an infection. It is a measure of the virus's capability of how frequently it can infect another same type of species (horizontal transmission). To determine the extent of the infectivity of the virus, an R_0 value was used. R_0 value is a measure for the average number of people who would contract a contagious disease from one person with that disease. Value more than one indicates the possibility of an outbreak or epidemic. The R_0 value was calculated using ordinary differential equations based on data obtained from contact tracing. This value is entirely subjective since it is highly dependent on the reporting rate of the disease. The R_0 for the coronavirus was calculated between 1.4 and 6.47. This means that one person can infect 1.4–6.47 persons. In addition, according to the most comprehensive and up-to-date calculations, the doubling rate of the coronavirus was 1.8 days as of March 2020. Value more than one indicates the possibility of an outbreak or epidemic.

The primary route of transmission of COVID-19 was found to be airborne droplets and direct contact. However, the fecal-oral transmission may occur since viral molecules were detected in the stool samples of pneumonia patients with gastrointestinal symptoms. Generally, children tend to be asymptomatic with the virus but are paramount vectors of COVID-19 transmission. This is because being asymptomatic means that these children do not display symptoms of the virus. Therefore, it becomes harder to track or make necessary precautions if children do not test for the presence of COVID-19.

The lethality of COVID-19 varies by age group. According to Dr. Bhattacharya, there is a 95% survival rate for people over age 70 infected with COVID-19. For people under age 70, the survival rate is 99.95%. He also states that for children, the flu is more deadly than

COVID-19. According to the CDC, as of August 2021, there have been more COVID-19 deaths than flu deaths among the American population.

2.0 Coronavirus: A Virological Perspective

1.2 Detection of the Coronavirus

There are three well-established methods to detect the COVID-19: (a) chest CT scan, (b) PCR, (c) viral gene sequencing. Some precursors to COVID-19 are decreased leukocyte (white blood cells), lymphocyte (lymph cells) and platelet (cells responsible for clotting) counts.

1.2.1 Chest CT Scan

The medical community recommends that all people suspected of COVID-19 take a chest CT scan in order to verify the presence of respiratory pathogens. Because the symptoms and target cells of COVID-19 are similar to that of viral pneumonia, the chest CT scan reveals similar results. For example, the CT examination reveals multiple patchy appearances (lobular and post-segmental consolidation), ground glass changes, and thickening of interlobular septa, also known as cobblestone changes. Generally, radiology is contraindicated when assessing the presence of COVID-19 in seniors because radiological disorders are more prevalent in the elderly.

2.1.2 PCR

Alternate forms of testing include the nucleic acid test, which is performed via PCR (polymerase chain reaction). In the polymerase chain reaction, there are short DNA sequences called primers that are created to select the portion of the DNA that is amplified. Once the primer binds, the temperature of the surrounding environment increases, and the primer complex becomes separated from the DNA itself. Then the temperature is cooled so that the primer can anneal itself. This results in the primer segments being cooled and the DNA being hardened. This process continues until millions and millions of copies are made. This process is common in the extraction step of COVID-19 testing. If one tests positive for COVID-19, then their sample (the chemicals contained in the swab) will contain certain sequences that are also present in COVID-19. If one tests negative, these target sequences will not be detected.

A detailed image of the PCR primer process can be found at https://www.genome.gov/genetics-glossary/Polymerase-Chain-Reaction. First, the new primer targets a chain of DNA and one copy is formed. This process happens at high temperatures. Then, these primer sequences form new strands based on complementary DNA base pairing. If the process is repeated, millions of DNA sequences can be generated, and biochemists can target this sequence when developing a vaccine.

2.1.3 Viral Gene Sequencing

This is the most accurate way of detecting the presence of COVID-19, primarily due to the fact that the researcher doesn't have to deal with the viral DNA being denatured in any way shape or form due to excessive heating. Just like PCR, the operon that the virus contains can be matched with the genetic code of your DNA in order to verifiably prove that one has the virus without any speculation needed. In order to extract the DNA of the respiratory tract cells, it is recommended that the swab test be performed. If researchers find that a section of DNA or RNA matches the genome of the virus, then it is concluded that one has tested positive for COVID-19.

1.3 Structure of the Coronavirus

The membrane of the COVID-19 virus has three different types of proteins: spike proteins, membrane proteins, and envelope proteins. Overall, the diameter of the virus (excluding the spike proteins is approximately 65–125 nanometers). The spike proteins bind to the ACE2 receptors, and the membrane proteins prevent the entry of substances into the intracellular space of the virus. The envelope proteins serve as a filter for substances that are permitted to permeate through the COVID-19 viral membrane. The nucleocapsid forms complexes with the virus's genomic RNA and interacts.

As mentioned in the introduction, the virus has spike proteins protruding from its membrane, which is why the virus family was named coronavirus. The virus binds to angiotensin-converting enzyme 2, which is a precursor for diabetes; this is why people with diabetes are especially prone to getting infected with COVID-19 (Monchatre-Leroy et al. 2017).

1.4 Replication

COVID-19 primarily enters the host via endocytosis and is only capable of replicating inside the host. Upon entering the host cell, COVID-19 releases its own genome and viral polymerase proteins. COVID-19 then uses the host cell's machinery to replicate its RNA-based genome. It then uses the host cell's machinery to create its own structural proteins via translation. The structural proteins, which are discussed in an earlier section, will combine with a nucleocapsid to form the mature virion. This replicated virus then escapes the host cell via exocytosis. These steps are displayed in the figure below:

COVID-19 uses the cell's machinery to protect itself from further degradation and destruction. For example, the virus uses the human cell's machinery in order to replicate itself. In addition, the virus uses the Golgi vesicle in the human cell to inherently provide membranous protection from immune cells (Monchatre-Leroy et al. 2017).

1.5 Mechanism of Replication

COVID-19 uses angiotensin-converting enzyme 2 (ACE2) receptor-binding motif (RBM) as a receptor like that of SARS-CoV. The angiotensin-converting-enzyme 2 motif is commonly found in type II alveolar cells. These type II alveolar cells produce and release surfactants, which increase lung compliance when breathing. What COVID-19 seeks to do is influence the function of these type II alveolar cells, thus decreasing surfactant production, which is why those severely affected by the coronavirus are diagnosed with acute respiratory distress syndrome since their lungs have trouble expanding when breathing.

It can be concluded that the virus is particularly infectious and lethal to older populations and Asian populations since Asian populations have a higher ACE2 expressing cell ratio than other ethnicities (Cao 2020). This phenomenon could also explain the proliferation of COVID-19 in China. In addition, it is also known that once people get older, their ACE2 expressing cell ratios increase, which could explain increased infectivity and lethality of COVID-19 in senior populations.

3. COVID Variants

Like all viral particles, COVID-19 evolves into different variants, based on the immunity of the human population in that region. There are generally three steps to the evolution of viruses. The first step happens during DNA or RNA replication. There is generally a mutation (error in DNA or RNA replication in which the replicated segment is not the same as the original segment) or polyploidy (error in replication in which multiple genomes are present within the capsid of the virus) present in the virus that enables the virus to survive the original medical treatment. As a result, the viruses that contain the genes or the polyploidy that enables them to survive traditional medical treatment survive, and those that do not contain the necessary genome die via natural selection. However, viruses have also found a way to transmit genetic information to other viruses so that they acquire immunity from traditional medical treatment as well. According to A T Still University, viruses exchange genetic information in three different ways: reassortment, polyploidy, and recombination.

3.1 Reassortment

Reassortment is defined as an exchange of nucleic acid segments between viruses with segmented genomes. This is the most common method in which viruses gain resistance or infectivity by altering their genome. Viruses share and exchange genetic information with each other, which promotes the resistance of the virus to medical treatments.

3.2 Polyploidy

The third and final way that viruses can evolve and gain resistance is by polyploidy. Polyploidy can happen with viruses from the same species or viruses from different species. Polyploidy is defined as the incorporation of more than one complete genome into the same virus capsid. A virus can incorporate genetic information of the virus of the same species or viruses from different species. When the virus incorporates information from viruses of different species, the phenomenon is referred to as heteroploidy or genotypic mixing. Polyploidy can increase the genetic variance of the virus, thus inherently making it resistant to a variety of environments.

3.3 Recombination

Recombination allows the virus to rearrange fragments of DNA and RNA by breaking them and then reuniting them. As a result, via transcription and translation, different proteins can be produced, therefore reducing the impact of original medical treatments on the virus. According to the NIH, beta coronaviruses are thought to primarily evolve via recombination.

According to the CDC, there were five notable variants in the United States as of August 2021. The B.1.1.7 variant is commonly referred to as the British variant. It was initially discovered in the United States in December 2020. The B.1.351 variant is commonly referred to as the South African variant and was discovered in the US in January 2021. The P1 variant, also commonly known as the Brazilian variant, was initially discovered in the US in January 2021. The last two variants, B.1.427 and B.1.429, were not discovered in other countries before they were discovered in the United States. In fact, these variants were initially discovered in California in February 2021. The delta variant was discovered in India in December 2020. As of August 2021, according to the CDC, these variants seem to spread more quickly than the original virus. The omicron variant emerged in

November 2121 as a more virulent strain with different symptoms and a much lower lethality.

In response to these variants, as well as many others found around the world, the CDC has provided a robust classification system regarding the threat of these variants. They have divided the categories into variants of interest, variants of concern, and variants of high consequence.

3.3.1 Variants of Interest

Variants of Interest usually have specific genetic markers that may affect receptor binding or reduce neutralization by antibodies generated from the previous infection. As a result, these variants may reduce the efficacy of traditional treatments against COVID-19. This means that some COVID-19 vaccines may not work as effectively in reducing the infectivity and severity of the variants. In order for the COVID-19 variant to be a variant of interest, the genetic difference between the original virus, and the variant must affect the transmission, immune cell resistance, diagnostics, or medicinal treatment of the virus. In addition, there also must be evidence that the genetic variance is a cause for the increased proportion of cases or uniquely clustered cases.

3.3.2 Variants of Concern

The criteria for variants of concern are just more stringent than the criteria for variants of interest. However, there are some glaring differences. For example, there must be evidence that the COVID-19 variant impacts diagnosis, treatments, or vaccines. The CDC spells out the following criteria for evidence. For example, the CDC explicitly states that in order to prove that the variant impacts diagnosis, treatments, or vaccines, there must be widespread interference with diagnostic test targets, Evidence of substantially decreased susceptibility to one or more classes of therapies must be demonstrated. Scientists must also demonstrate evidence that the variant has significantly decreased neutralization by antibodies generated during previous infection or vaccination.

3.3.3 Variants of High Consequence

For a COVID-19 variant to be considered a variant of high consequence, there must be evidence that medical countermeasures have not significantly reduced the effectiveness of the virus. Despite providing adequate medical countermeasures if the variant demonstrates a significant reduction in vaccine effectiveness, a disproportionately high number of vaccine breakthrough cases or low vaccine-induced protection against severe disease. As of August 2021, there are no COVID-19 variants that are considered variants of high consequences, which is an indication that the medical countermeasures have been effective at preventing the infectivity and curbing the lethality of COVID-19.

4.0 Vaccine Generation

All in all, there have been 9 total frontiers of vaccine development for viruses: whole inactivated, live attenuated, split inactivated, synthetic peptide, virus-like particles, DNA or RNA, recombinant subunits, recombinant bacterial vectors, and recombinant viral vectors. Of these nine total frontiers, only seven of them were considered legitimate vaccine platforms for COVID-19. Each frontier, except for DNA and RNA vaccine has some precedent of administration and efficacy. The figure depicting the vaccine frontiers that were considered for the COVID-19 vaccine is shown in Table 1 (Monchatre-Leroy 2017).

Table 1. Advantages and Disadvantages of Different Vaccine Platforms

Vaccine Platform	Advantages	Disadvantages	Clinical Examples
Whole inactivated virus vaccine	Stronger immune response; safer than live attenuated	Potential epitope alteration by inactivation process	Typhoid, cholera, hepititis A, plague, rabies, influenza, polio (salk)
Live attenuated virus vaccine	Stronger immune response; preservation of native antigen, mimicking natural infection	Risk of residual virulence, especially for immuno-Calmette-Guerin (BCG), compromised people	Measles, mumps, polio (sabin), rota virus, yellow fever, bacillus, rubella, varicella
Viral vector vaccine	Stronger immune immune response preservation of native antigen, mimicking natural infection	More complicated manufacturing process; risk of genomic integration; response dampened by preexisting immunity against vector	Ebola virus
Subunit vaccine	Safe and well tolerated adjuvant of conjugate to increase immunogenicity	Lower immunogenicity requirement of pneumoniae, *Haemophilus influenza type b*	Pertusis, Influenza, *Streptococcus,*
Viral-like particle vaccine	Safe and well tolerated; mimicking native virus conformation	Lower immunogenicity; more complicated manufacturing process	Hepatitis B virus, human papilloma-virus
DNA vaccine	Safe and well tolerated; stable under room temp; highly adaptable to new pathogen; native antigen expression	Lower immunogenicity; Difficult administration route; Risk of genomic integration	N/A
RNA vaccine	Safe and well tolerated; highly adaptable to new pathogen; native antigen expression	Lower immunogenicity; requires low temp storage and transportation; potential risk of RNA-induced interferon response	N/A

Note: Different vaccine platform approaches
considered in making the COVID-19 vaccine

The whole inactivated virus vaccine approach has been proven to elicit a stronger immune response by diluting the potency of the virus in patients with typhoid, cholera, hepatitis A, plague, rabies, influenza, and polio. The live attenuated virus vaccine platform elicits a stronger immune response by mimicking the natural infection. With this mode of vaccine development, there is a risk of spreading the natural infection to other hosts. The live attenuated vaccine platform has been used when developing the measles, mumps, polio, rotavirus, yellow fever, rubella, and varicella vaccines with high levels of efficacy. The viral vaccine platform uses a similar vaccine approach but has less viral infectivity than the live attenuated viral vaccine platform. This platform has commonly been used when developing the Ebola vaccine. The development of protein subunit vaccines may sound complex, but it is simpler than that of the whole virus and viral vector vaccines. Protein subunit vaccines consist of viral antigenic fragments produced by recombinant protein techniques. The protein subunit vaccines are also significantly less lethal than the whole virus vaccines. However, a primary drawback of these types of vaccines is that the low immunogenicity; the vaccine may not elicit the desired extent of the immune response as other types of vaccines. Also, one may need to take another shot of the protein subunit vaccine later in their life because the immunogenicity is so low. The virus-like particle vaccine seeks to mimic the structure of the virus but the particle itself does not contain viral DNA or RNA. With the COVID-19 vaccine, scientists can mimic the arrangement of the spike, membrane and envelope proteins of the COVID-19 virus, and this can elicit an adequate immune response in humans. This kind of vaccine platform has been used in the development of the HPV vaccine and the hepatitis B virus. The DNA vaccine platform is safe and well-tolerated, but the conditioned immune response may wear out over time and a supplemental dose may be required. The same advantages and disadvantages are present with the RNA vaccine.

4.1 Vaccine Efficacy

As of August 2021, there are five main types of vaccines in circulation worldwide. Of these five vaccines, only three of them are FDA approved for emergency use. The most effective of these FDA-approved vaccines is the Pfizer-BioNTech vaccine. The Pfizer-BioNTech vaccine was approved by the FDA on December 11, 2020. According to yalemedicine.org, the Pfizer-BioNTech vaccine is an mRNA vaccine that is 95% effective. As stated in the previous chapter and the table above, one of the advantages of this kind of vaccine is that it is highly adaptable to new pathogens. In fact, according to yalemedicine.org, the Pfizer vaccine was found to be 95% effective against the British and South African variants of the virus, which is why the Pfizer-BioNTech vaccine is effective against a majority of COVID-19 variants. Furthermore, with the Pfizer-BioNTech vaccine, it is required to be stored in cold temperatures because in the presence of room temperature, the RNA of the virus may get degraded, and the virus is no longer effective. The Pfizer-BioNTech vaccine allows the human body to make its own spike protein and then elicit an immune response against the spike protein.

The second vaccine that was approved by the FDA was the Moderna vaccine. The Moderna vaccine was approved on December 18, 2020. Like the Pfizer-BioNTech vaccine, the Moderna vaccine is also an mRNA vaccine and has similar drawbacks to the Pfizer-BioNTech vaccine. There is a requirement for cold temperature storage. However, the Moderna vaccine is less effective with older populations than the Pfizer vaccine. The Pfizer vaccine has 94.1% efficacy for people over 65 and the Moderna vaccine is 86% effective for people over 65.

The third vaccine that was approved by the FDA was the Johnson and Johnson vaccine. The Johnson & Johnson vaccine was approved on February 7, 2021. However, the FDA only approved the

Johnson & Johnson vaccine for emergency purposes. This was because there were six incidences of blood clotting in women from ages 18 to 48, occurring 6 to 13 days after vaccination. On April 23, 2021, the CDC voted to end the pause of the Johnson & Johnson vaccine under the condition that there would be a mandatory label stating that blood clots may occur. Johnson & Johnson is also recommended for people 18 and older. The storage requirements for Johnson & Johnson are not as restrictive since the vaccine is a viral vector vaccine. More information about viral vector vaccines can be found in the table about the advantages and disadvantages of different vaccine platforms.

There are two vaccines that are still not FDA-approved. These are the Oxford-AstraZeneca vaccine and the Novavax vaccine. As of August 2021, The Oxford-AstraZeneca vaccine is being distributed in the UK and some other countries due to the low cost of production. Also, the Oxford-AstraZeneca vaccine can be stored at room temperature for six months, so transport is easier.

The Oxford-AstraZeneca vaccine is proven to be 76% effective at reducing the risk of symptomatic disease after vaccination. AstraZeneca also claims that the vaccine is 85% effective at preventing COVID-19 for people over 65. However, the NIAID (National Institute of Allergies and Infectious Diseases) expressed concern about the new data that AstraZeneca reported to the FDA. The AstraZeneca vaccine is administered in two doses. The second dose must be taken 4 to 12 weeks after the first dose.

The Novavax vaccine uses a different vaccine platform than all of the other vaccines. Novavax uses a protein adjuvant platform, which means that the Novavax vaccine already contains the mimicked spike protein, instead of containing the genetic information required to make the spike protein. The vaccine has to be administered twice, and the second dose must be three weeks apart from the first dose. According to the vaccine classifications previously discussed, the Novavax vaccine can be described as a subunit vaccine. In addition, the spike protein exists as a nanoparticle so that there is no consequence if the immune system fails to detect the spike protein. The Novavax phase 2B clinical trials revealed that the vaccine was 86.3% effective against the British variant and 55.4% effective against the B.1.351 variant for HIV-negative patients.

5.0 Vaccine Distribution and Administration Challenges and Approaches

5.1 Storage of Vaccine

As discussed in the vaccines section of this chapter, each vaccine has different storage requirements. As a result, there have been challenges in the transport of vaccines.

5.1.1 Pfizer Vaccine

According to Pfizer, their brand's vaccine must be stored in temperatures of -70 degrees Celsius with a margin of error of 10 degrees Celsius. They also cite that the vaccine cannot be refrozen. They cite three possible storage options: Ultra-low temperature freezers, Pfizer's own thermal shipper, and the refrigeration units available in hospitals. Of these three recommended methods of storage, only two are feasible for transport and the refrigeration units in hospitals are only capable of reaching temperatures of 2–8 degrees Celsius. The ultra-low temperature freezers can extend the life of the Pfizer vaccine up to six months. The thermal shippers must be replenished with dry ice every five days since dry ice sublimes in the environment of the cooler.

5.1.2 Moderna Vaccine

According to the CDC, the storage requirements for the Moderna vaccine storage are the following: the vaccine will arrive frozen between –25 °C and –15 °C and needs to be stored at the same temperature. After defrosting, the vaccine may be thawed in the refrigerator or at room temperature. The vaccine must be refrigerated at 2 °C to 8 °C for 2 hours and 30 minutes. The un-punctured vials may be kept between 8 °C and 25 °C for up to 12 hours. Thawed vaccines cannot be refrozen. Vaccine vials may be stored in the refrigerator between 2 °C and 8 °C for up to 30 days before vials are punctured. Furthermore, after 30 days, any remaining vials should be removed from the refrigerator and discarded following manufacturer and jurisdiction guidance on proper disposal.

5.1.3 Oxford-AstraZeneca Vaccine:

The British government has created the following requirements for the storage of the Oxford-AstraZeneca vaccine; it must be stored at temperatures of 2–8 degrees Celsius, the vaccine must not freeze, and after the first dose is withdrawn, the vaccine should be used as soon as possible and within six hours.

6.0 General Conclusions

There are clear obstacles of the administration of the vaccines due to their stringent storage requirements. Of the three vaccines discussed above, the Oxford-AstraZeneca has the least stringent storage requirements since the vaccine can be stored infinitely. However, the time between opening the first dose and administration is the most stringent of the three vaccines since the vaccine must be administered within six hours from opening the shipment. In terms of storage, the

Pfizer vaccine is the most stringent as it requires storage temperatures that can only be achieved by surrounding the shipment in dry ice or liquid nitrogen. This may also be factored in the cost of the Pfizer vaccine. With all three vaccines, thawed vaccines cannot be refrozen.

6.1 Affordability of the Vaccine

The cost of the COVID-19 vaccine varies from country to country. Governments are primarily using taxpayer money to buy doses of the vaccine from Big Pharma. According to the BMJ, the US is paying $19.50 per dose of the Pfizer vaccine, whereas the European Union is paying $14.70 per dose. For the Moderna vaccine, the US is paying less than the European Union (the US is paying $15 per dose and the EU is paying $18 per dose). The reason the pricing is less for the EU than the US for the Pfizer vaccine is because the EU funded the development of the Pfizer vaccine and therefore it is willing to charge EU governments less for the vaccine itself. The same logic applies to the Moderna vaccine.

6.2 Licensing Agreements between Countries and Manufacturers

An important issue with the administration of the COVID-19 vaccine is the licensing agreements between the companies and foreign nations that didn't play a role in the manufacturing of the vaccine. As mentioned in the affordability section, the Pfizer and Moderna vaccines are being bought by the US and European Union countries relatively freely. The United Kingdom has its own AstraZeneca vaccine that is funded by its own taxpayers. Therefore, there haven't been many licensing disputes between these three factions since each side has its own taxpayer-funded vaccine. However, there are countries that do not possess such resources to make their own efficacious COVID-19 vaccine. As a result, AstraZeneca has formed licensing agreements with the Serum Institute of India, Gavi the Vaccine Alliance, and the Coalition for Epidemic Preparedness Innovations (CEPI). According to AstraZeneca, AstraZeneca had reached a 750-million-dollar agreement with the CEPI and Gavi to support the manufacturing, procurement, and distribution of 300 million doses of the vaccine in June 2020. AstraZeneca has also agreed with the Serum Institute of India to provide 400 million doses to middle and low-income Indian citizens.

As of August 2021, in terms of providing developing countries with the resources to develop their own vaccine, a TRIPS waiver has been proposed. The TRIPS waiver would allow companies in other countries to use the same methodology without any legal liability that Pfizer and Moderna used to develop their vaccines. This would help vaccine administration in these countries greatly. This protection from liability would last at least ten years. Specifically, this TRIPS waiver would help countries like India with robustly producing and distributing the vaccine in a world health crisis. Key proponents of the TRIPS waiver include India, South Africa, and the African CDC. In India and African countries, there have been long lines and excessive demand for the COVID vaccine. Unfortunately, the supply of the vaccine doesn't meet the demand for the vaccine. An important issue with the TRIPS waiver is that Pfizer and Moderna would have to sacrifice their intellectual property rights and give this information out to foreign companies. In turn, they cannot sue for infringements on intellectual property. This skews the demand for the COVID-19 vaccine in the international market, which deprives pharma companies of their revenue and irritates shareholders. According to *Reuters*, Dr. Amesh Adalija attests that this patent waiver results in the expropriation of the intellectual property of Pfizer and Moderna, which is unethical and unfair. Bill Gates also opposes the TRIPS waiver due to intellectual property protection issues.

6.3. Handling the Side Effects of the Vaccine

According to the CDC, common adverse side effects of the COVID-19 vaccine are tiredness, headache, muscle pain, chills, fever, and nausea. This is primarily due to the immune response to spike protein production. It is also known that the side effects are exacerbated when the second shot is taken. In addition, myocarditis is a common side effect of the mRNA COVID-19 vaccine. According to the CDC, this is a common effect of the mRNA vaccine platform. As of June 2021, federal health officials reported 226 cases of myocarditis among vaccinated individuals in the United States. They were also investigating 250 additional reports at that time. The CDC recommends the handling of adverse COVID-19 vaccine reactions just like they handle other adverse reactions: there is a vaccine adverse reporting system (VAERS) where people can complain about the wrongful administration of the vaccine and its associated side effects. In the emergency rooms, the treatments indicated for the side effects will be performed in terms of handling the adverse effects of COVID-19.

6.4 Long-Term Effects of Vaccines

Like any other vaccine, in the long term, the efficacy of the current vaccine may decrease due to the fact that like microorganisms, viruses evolve rather rapidly. Therefore, the drugs that had once worked against COVID-19 will not work because the virus would have mutated an enzyme that degrades the vaccine before it acts on the virus. There are already serious questions about the efficacy of the current vaccine on the delta variant of COVID-19. As a result, the medical community will once again have to create vaccines that are more efficacious against these variants of COVID-19. Generally, the way that the medical community handles this (especially with the influenza vaccines) is that they try to predict the subsequent mutation that the virus will then take and then target the characteristics of that mutation. When these predictions become incorrect, there may be another lockdown and additional precautions may need to be taken prior to vaccine development.

References

Achaiah, N. C., Subbarajasetty, S. B., and Shetty, R. M. 2020. "Ro and Re of COVID-19: Can we predict when the pandemic outbreak will be contained?" *Indian Journal of Critical Care Medicine,* 24 (11) (November 24): 1125–1127. https://doi. org/10.5005%2Fjp-journals-10071-23649

Anand, P., and Stahel, V. P. 2021. "The safety of COVID-19 mRNA vaccines: a review." *Patient Safety in Surgery,* 15 (1): 1–9. https:// doi.org/10.1186/s13037-021-00291-9

Bhattacharya, J., and Gupta, S. 2020. "How to End Lockdowns next month." *The Wall Street Journal* (December 17). https://www.wsj. com/articles/how-to-end-lockdowns-next-month-11608230214

Cao, Y., Li, L., Feng, Z., Wan, S., Huang, P., Sun, X., Wen, F., Huang, X., Ning, G., and Wang, W. 2020. "Comparative genetic analysis of the novel coronavirus (2019-ncov/sars-cov-2) receptor ACE2 in different populations." *Cell Discovery,* 6 (11) (February 24). https://doi.org/10.1038/s41421-020-0147-1

Centers for Disease Control and Prevention. 2021. *SARS-CoV-2 Variant Classifications and Definitions* (October 4). Retrieved November

27, 2021. https://www.cdc.gov/coronavirus/2019-ncov/variants/variant-info.html

Cueno, M. E., and Imai, K. 2021. "Structural comparison of the SARS-CoV 2 spike protein relative to other human-infecting coronaviruses." *Frontiers in Medicine* (January 14). https://doi.org/10.3389/fmed.2020.594439

Kaplan, D. A., and Wehrwein, P. 2021. The price tags on the COVID-19 vaccines. *Managed Healthcare Executive,* 31 (3) (March 15). https://www.managedhealthcareexecutive.com/view/the-price-tags-on-the-covid-19-vaccines

Li, Y. D., Chi, W. Y., Su, J. H., Ferrall, L., Hung, C. F., and Wu, T. C. 2020. "Coronavirus vaccine development: from SARS and MERS to COVID-19." *Journal of Biomedical Science, 27* (1), 1–23. https://doi.org/10.1186/s12929-020-00695-2

Monchatre-Leroy, E., Boué, F., Boucher, J.-M., Renault, C., Moutou, F., Ar Gouilh, M., and Umhang, G. 2017. "Identification of alpha and Beta coronavirus in wildlife species in France: Bats, rodents, rabbits, and hedgehogs." *Viruses, 9* (12) (November 29): 364. https://doi.org/10.3390/v9120364

National Center for Immunization and Respiratory Diseases (NCIRD), Division of Viral Diseases. 2021. "Science brief: Emerging SARS-CoV-2 variants" (January 28). National Library of Medicine. https://pubmed.ncbi.nlm.nih.gov/34009774/

National Center for Immunization and Respiratory Diseases (US) Disease Control and Prevention. 2021. "About variants of the virus that causes COVID-19. Centers for Disease Control and Prevention" (April 2). https://stacks.cdc.gov/view/cdc/104698

National Human Genome Research Institute. 2021. *Polymerase chain reaction (PCR)* (September 14). https://www.genome.gov/genetics-glossary/Polymerase-Chain-Reaction

Santos, A. F., Gaspar, P. D., and de Souza, H. J. 2021. "Refrigeration of COVID-19 VACCINES: Ideal Storage Characteristics, energy efficiency and environmental impacts of Various Vaccine Options." *Energies, 14* (7): 1849. https://doi.org/10.3390/en14071849

Shalal, A., Mason, J., Lawder, D. 2021. "U.S. reverses stance, backs giving poorer countries access to COVID vaccine patents." *Reuters* (May 5). Retrieved November 27, 2021. Reuters.com

Widakuswara, P. 2021. "Biden agrees to waive COVID-19 vaccine patents, but it's still complicated." *Voice of America News* (May 5). https://www.voanews.com/a/covid-19-pandemic_biden-agrees-waive-covid-19-vaccine-patents-its-still-complicated/6205485.html

Glossary of Terms

airborne. The term used to refer to the aerial transmission of a virus or bacterial infection.

asymptomatic. It is when a person has an infection but does not display the associated symptoms of the infection.

capsid. The membrane of the virus.

coronavirus. A virus whose outer membrane comprises spike proteins that protrude out of the membrane.

efficacy. The effectiveness of something.

endocytosis. A process where substances are transported into the cell. It involves membrane fusion of the vesicle in which substances are being transported and the extracellular membrane itself.

epidemic. A widespread occurrence of an infectious disease in a community at a particular time.

epidemiological: Pertaining to a widespread occurrence of an infectious disease in a community at a particular time.

etiology. Causes or set of causes of something.

enzyme. A substance that catalyzes a biological reaction.

glycoproteins. Proteins on the periphery of the virus that bind to the receptor of a human or animal cell.

nucleocapsid. The RNA and nuclear membrane inside of the virus.

polyploidy. A phenomenon where there are more than a pair of the same chromosome (triplet, quartet, quintet, etc.).

polymerase chain reaction. A process involving the creation of new DNA in which primers are cleaved and then new copies are created.

reassortment. Exchange of nucleic acid segments between viruses with segmented genomes.

recombination. A process of transmitting a favorable genotype from one microorganism to another, only common in bacteria and viruses.

sublimation. A phase transition from solid phase to a gas phase.

CHAPTER 9

Quantum Computers—Using Change Management to Study the Pandemic

by Nicolas M. Casati and Kevin M. Sorbello

Abstract

The pandemic has multiple consequences, many of which can be addressed through change management. The primary consequence of the pandemic was a global public health crisis, which has been tackled with vaccines by Pfizer, Moderna, Johnson & Johnson, and more vaccines that may be developed to close the gap between the current pandemic and future variants. The issues created by the pandemic are emblematic of the ever-changing internal (corporate) and external (policy) challenges that need to be addressed by all levels of management.

A review of the COVID-19 history shows a rollout of a functioning vaccine in record time can be achieved by simultaneously testing the efficacy of multiple vaccine candidates. However, trial vaccines may be found inefficient or less effective than anticipated and the public's perception based on a variety of cultural biases could delay the trials or eventual deployment of the vaccines. This is where more expansive and inclusive change management techniques must be developed and employed.

The most significant impact to change management could be the result of introducing quantum computers into the algorithms, vaccine development, and complex social adaptations where conventional computers are overtaxed with the span of information and its often-conflicting nature.

Keywords: Pandemic, quantum computer, change management, algorithms

1. Introduction

The global state of affairs has been shaken to its core and continues to be rearranged through change management since the COVID-19 pandemic changed the status quo. When we manage a change project, our human nature inclines us to view the world in terms of an aesthetic ratio, commonly known as the golden ratio (a ratio equal to 1.618). Although perhaps unconsciously aware of this tendency, scholars as far back as Pythagoras and Euclid recognized patterns in nature. The golden ratio is derived from the Fibonacci series (1, 1, 2, 3, 5, 8, etc.), and in mathematics, it is obtained by dividing 8 by 5 to get 1.618. The observed sequence is most seen in nature where plants and trees show that pattern in optimizing leaf placement for maximum photosynthetic exposure to light. Nature organizes and manages change according to the golden ratio, and we tend to do the same. The pandemic, leading senior government leaders to transition related an environment where reactionary and progressive politics prepared polarizing agendas. In December 2018, the U.S. conservative electorate signed HR 6227, the National Quantum Initiative Act into law because technical competitiveness was the priority in the collective change management mind.

The COVID-19 pandemic required reprioritization of intended actions, resulting in an accelerated COVID-19 vaccine development effort to address manufacturing challenges called Operation Warp Speed (OWS). The intent of this initiative, a partnership between the Departments of Health and Human Services (HHS) and Defense (DoD) was to accelerate the development and production of an effective vaccine by adopting several strategies to accelerate development while mitigating risk (US GAO 2021). The OWS selected vaccine candidates using different mechanisms to stimulate an immune response (mRNA and vector). The same curve tool used for tracking COVID-19 patient samples to calculate how many doses of vaccine to produce was also used to determine the quantum mechanics of a quantum computer. The curve jargon used in mass media today such as: "flattening the curve," standard deviations, and the population versus sample mean came from Gottfried Leibniz born in the seventeenth century. Much like vaccine development's highly standardized operating procedures (temperature, pressure, etc.), a quantum computer "operates in niobium qubit, it has to be kept below 0.15 degrees Kelvin, within a magnetic field 50 thousand times less than Earth's and under 10 billion times less pressure than the outside" (Casati 2020, 23). The democratization of machines specialized maintaining inclement temperature/pressure conditions for vaccine preservation is favorable to the future widespread of technological capability necessary to keep a quantum computer working properly. At the beginning of the pandemic, companies capable of vaccine development were contracted to start large-scale manufacturing during clinical trials, combining clinical trials, or running them concurrently.

Financial initiatives were initially more focused on Operation Warp Speed change management initiatives with Pfizer and Moderna's spike mRNA vaccines. The first shock wave was healthcare-related due to the emergence of COVID-19, but a second shock wave might be a negative financial impact on the economy, leading to "negative interest rates territory, which was the case for some 30-year German bonds" and high "unemployment and inflation" (Casati 2020, 125). Meanwhile, Jansen (Johnson and Johnson) and AstraZeneca used a spike gene method with a non-replicating virus, and Sanofi/GSK and Novavax used a fully formed spike protein of SARS-CoV 2.

In spite of polarized politics often caricaturized as exceedingly capitalist, money hungry, Republicans versus welfare state Democrats, the result of government contracts under both Republicans and Democrats resulted in elevating Pfizer Inc. stock from $36 to $54 per share, and Moderna from $19 to $449 per share by mid-2021. However, the introduction of quantum computing could possibly detect any complex algorithmic financial manipulation schemes not identifiable with classical computers.

2. New Change Management Based on Quantum Computers

The pandemic has multiple consequences, many of which can be addressed through change management. The primary consequence of the pandemic was a global public health crisis, which has been tackled with vaccines by Pfizer, Moderna, Johnson & Johnson, and more vaccines that may be developed to close the gap between the current pandemic and future variants. The issues created by the pandemic are emblematic of the ever-changing internal (corporate) and external (policy) challenges that need to be addressed by all levels of management.

A review of recent history shows a rollout of a functioning vaccine in record time can be achieved by simultaneously testing the efficacy of multiple vaccine candidates. However, trial vaccines may be found inefficient or less effective than anticipated and the public's perception based on a variety of cultural biases could delay the trials or eventual deployment of the vaccines. This is where more expansive and inclusive change management techniques must be developed and employed.

The most significant impact to change management could be the result of introducing algorithms into quantum computers used for vaccine development, and complex social adaptations where conventional computers are overtaxed with the span of information and its often-conflicting nature.

Quantum computers, a technology still under development (CBInsights 2021), could significantly shorten the time required to develop effective vaccines, respond to shifts in social norms, perceptions, and expectations, and provide a more comprehensive analysis of a quickly evolving social, political, and natural environment. Using quantum computers could provide the effective change management tool necessary to simultaneously address internal and external shifts while building an optimal infrastructure for the logistical distribution of the vaccine.

Quantum computing is still in development, and some detractors suggest a functional or practical quantum computer is virtually impossible to create due to random hardware errors (Kak 2019; Edmunds 2021) posited that quantum computing technology must overcome the limitations imposed by errors affecting quantum devices. However, Google, Microsoft, and PsiQuantum have made technological progress in bringing quantum computers from theory to practice. In 2019 Google used a 53-qubit chip to solve a problem in just a few minutes that would have taken a classical computer 10,000 years to complete. Just over a year later, China claimed it had performed a calculation in 200 seconds that would have taken a classical computer 2.5 billion years. IBM plans to create a 1,000-qubit computer by 2023, and Microsoft-backed PsiQuantum plans to build a 1 million-qubit computer within the next five years (CBInsights 2021).

The secret to the quantum computer's lightning speed lies in its architecture. Classical computers use transistors that represent a 0 or a 1, depending on whether they are turned on or off. Quantum computers, on the other hand, calculate with qubits which exist as a 0 and a 1 at the same time. A classical computer's power increases in a 1:1 relationship with the number of transistors while a quantum computer's power increases exponentially with the number of qubits (Wang et al. 2021). Classical computers have low error rates and can operate at room temperature while quantum computers have high error rates and need to be kept in an ultra-cold environment, at least with our current informatics technology. The temperature was first measured by thermometers with a centigrade scale described in Casati (1992). However, while classical computers are very effective at processing everyday calculations, quantum computers have a significant advantage for optimizing problems, data analysis, and simulations, especially in complex, often contradictory situations. As such, a universal quantum computer can be used to solve a wider range of simulations and problems (Dubé et al. 2020). While new algorithms are being developed, Shor's algorithm for factoring large numbers is the current standard for encryption breaking, and Grover's algorithm is best used for accelerated searching through massive sets of data (Casati 2021b).

The reality is that quantum computing proponents currently outnumber those who claim the impracticality of creating a functional and reliable machine. For example, PsiQuantum, a company focused on quantum computer development, has $278.5M in disclosed funding. Cambridge Quantum Computing, a well-funded startup company, has raised $95M from investors such as IBM, Honeywell, and others. Microsoft and Amazon have partnered with IonQ and Rigeti to eventually produce quantum computers for Azure and AWS. Other tech giants like Google are heavily invested in quantum computing startups such as IonQ, ProteinQure, and Kuano. Google is not alone in such investments. Honeywell, Alibaba, Intel, and a host of others have invested substantial sums in their own development and those of other startups. Such excitement and investments by such leading technology companies are an indication of their belief in the viability of creating universal quantum computers.

3. How Quantum Computers Would Aid in the Development of Vaccines

The development, testing, and distribution of vaccines currently follow a traditional process, where basic science research traditionally happens before development and clinical testing, ultimately followed by its mass production and distribution. Each process is inherently time-consuming and subject to current limitations of change management. However, government reaction to the pandemic resulted in a global economic crisis created by mandated shutdowns and lockdowns.

The unsustainability of such a situation forced vaccine research, clinical testing, mass production, and logistical distribution to work simultaneously within a single change management framework. Change management based on standard operating procedures is less effective under these circumstances, requiring review and revision of the previous models. However, the basics of change management theory are applicable and adaptable if properly applied. For example, the standard operating procedures of hand hygiene practiced by health care and food service workers are widely accepted and as such, more readily adaptable to the public to limit the spread of the virus. The same holds true for change management standards.

Researchers and developers can follow several protocols simultaneously if the standards are explained and handled with effective change management techniques. The traditional barriers between the three silos of research/development, mass production, and logistical distribution were removed by the need for expedited delivery of an effective vaccine, all under the adaptive elements of change management. The resulting new normal is one based on the need for adaptive change management; a change management-centric model that accepts the need for managing continuous change across multiple areas.

4. Implications of Developing and Applying Quantum Computers

The development and application of quantum computing can ensure oversight of large-scale spending provided in complex situations, especially when the time required for decisions is shorted due to the impact of the situation. Investing in quantum computing ultimately protects the economy while assisting change management development and adaptations toward future developments and the efficient deployment of treatments to all potential or actual pandemic victims.

Pandemics in general can be studied using future quantum computers and change management tools. Change management, which is the crux of this chapter, revolves around the science of learning. According to Barrow et al. (2017), "Two-thirds of all change projects fail for many reasons, such as poor planning, unmotivated staff, deficient communication, or excessively frequent changes" (Barrow et al., 2017). Change management needs good communication and assets like future quantum computers and a good staff to face the challenges resulting from a crisis such as a pandemic. Change management depends on a manager's experience, training in computers, a good team, and the wisdom associated with how best to use these resources.

Using oriental wisdom as a guide, the seven kinds of ultimate realities noted by Sridhar and Nagendra (2018) could theoretically be analyzed by future quantum computers and help with pandemics in terms of change management. A selection of these seven realities, only substance (dravya) or *essence* and *action* or motion (karma) are of interest here. Karma, in this case, refers to action, not the sum of a person's action in this and previous states of existence. Change management is in the realm of a human desire to improve the *substance* by *action*, and quantum computers could potentially address and advance research on pandemics in ways superior to conventional computing or thinking, or simply working harder.

The idea of hard work has been previously studied in *Rerum Novarum* by Pope Leo XIII and *The Wealth of Nations* by Adam Smith. There has recently been a change in the economy of work. This new economy of work further developed with the arrival of the pandemic because more and more people began conducting business from home. Working from home allowed virtual and remote workers to spend their time more productively, so the concept of working harder was replaced with working more efficiently and productively.

This shift, however, did not affect the business model used by the ultra-wealthy billionaire class selling services through stockbrokers to the upper-middle-class although the pandemic provided a new market in medicine that ushered in a unique opportunity for exponential wealth generation by proxy (as we saw with dramatic increases in Pfizer and

Moderna stock prices). The methods of wealth growth, however, are not always detectable at first glance.

5. Change Management

The complexity of change management during a pandemic, where biological sciences are developing at such a rapid rhythm that quantum chemistry algorithms will soon outpace informatics, create a situation where even quantum computers may be unable to solve these future problems (Xu and Ye 2020). Niccolo Machiavelli's understanding of the problem of change would be very different today due to the advent of machines like the quantum computer and the rapidity of change during a pandemic in general (Gill 2002). Machiavelli pointed out the difficulty and risk involved in implementing change due to a systemic resistance to change and a lack of commitment to it in his book *The Prince* (Gill 2002). The resistance to change and the lack of commitment are both exacerbated by conflicting and confusing information put out by politically and economically biased information presented during a pandemic. Analyzing and evaluating the validity of information, in addition to reading the perceptions and will of the people, cannot be effectively accomplished with classical computers. Powerful quantum computing, however, may help to alleviate the confusion, doubt, distrust, and angst felt by the general population by helping to develop better, more effective change management plans. Andrew Mayo stated, "Our organizations are littered with the debris . . . of yesterday's [change] initiatives" (Gill 2002, 307). Effective change management requires better, more informed planning and motivated staff (Barrow et al. 2017). Taking into account a wider range of variables is beyond conventional computing power and suggests the use of quantum computers that can more holistically address the complexities involved with change management during a pandemic.

There is a definite lack of resources and know-how and incompatible corporate policies and practices when it comes to dealing with pandemics (Gill 2002). It is paramount that researchers use the lessons learned from the latest pandemic to find better ways of addressing the challenges of future pandemics. Vermeiren (2021) argued an event such as worldwide influenza may be best described as an accident, which is controllable, while human death is considered essential and cannot be bent to our will. The accidental nature can be controlled through medical research. According to Gill (2002), if a relationship is external to what I am, then it can be measured by a quantum computer when a change management plan is drawn up.

6. Leadership and Change

There are special management techniques for which the umbrella term *change management* leads to different scenarios such as pandemics management or quantum computer research and development (Lauer 2010). Lauer noted that the "implementation of change is dependent on the active support of the employees" and "everyone has their own needs, ideas and experiences, some of which do not conform to the established corporate structure" (3). Lauer further indicated the three parties affected by change management are "individuals, the corporate structures, and the corporate culture" (3), and Casati (2021a) suggested corporate structure and culture can be assisted by future quantum computers.

There are different approaches to change management. External change can usually be measured using an instrument such as a computer or quantum computer (Lauer 2010). The requirement for such change can be caused by the market environment, politics, technology, ecology, or the economy (Lauer 2010). Internal changes are related to human development, sequence of growth, crisis, and higher maturity (Lauer 2010). In addition to external and internal changes, psychologists argue people avoid or devalue information that contradicts their previous attitude, and this is characterized by avoidance of cognitive dissonance (Lauer 2010). Facing future pandemics and addressing conflicting information, recommendations, and mandates could be an example of cognitive dissonance. The paradox is that managers who depend on adapting to a changing environment that allows business to grow (the ledger) also advance rational cost arguments not to change (Lauer 2010). The resistance to change from employees, especially the implementing employees and their managers is ubiquitous (Lauer 2010). Archibong and Ibrahim (2021) stressed the impact change management could have on employee performance and the need to properly tailor the change in context with the environment, culture, and makeup of the employees involved. In the case of quantum computer developments or pandemic vaccines, the effects of counterproductive resistance are to be avoided because it could result in a snowball effect of even greater resistance (Lauer 2010). The review of change management studies indicates those involved in the change process always need orientation about goals in order to maintain motivation during the course of the change to ensure sustainable success (Lauer 2010).

Lewin's *Field Theory on Social Change* demonstrated that "drivers of social change" are "applicable for business management settings" which could be assisted by quantum computers (Rosca 2020, 1). Lewin also had a strong interest in the nature and causes of social conflicts and how they can be approached with change management theory (Lewin 1997). Shuman et al. (2013) stated there are different types of valences which are based on appraisals of (un) pleasantness, goal obstructiveness, and conduciveness. Hayes (2018) had a different approach, arguing that change management was a way to transform organizations to maintain or improve their effectiveness, such as furthering research to prepare for future pandemics or developing quantum computers (Hayes 2018). Hayes (2018) posited that efficiency sustainment in resource usage while achieving company objectives propels organizational effectiveness (Hayes 2018). Hayes's (2018) approach to change management is different because he saw across its boundary to the external world as a key determinant to the process of change management (Hayes 2018).

7. Response to Vaccines Using Quantum Computers

Change management has been affected by COVID-19 in many ways, and the pandemic is causing risks and disruptions in most supply chains, which could be mitigated or avoided with the introduction of quantum computers (Hoek 2020). It has been posited that change involved in responding to risks will take time, and it is important for many companies to invest in quantum computing as a way to address the complexities associated with future pandemics (Hoek 2020). Change management will involve the eventual use of quantum computers as well as a different approach to the threats of future pandemics. Hoek (2020) argued quantum computers could accelerate the learning needed in a cross-functional engagement designed to address supply chain and vaccine development issues which currently take an extended period to be resolved.

Bhattacharyya (2020) posited that organizational change is either transactional or transformational, either of which can be assisted by future quantum computers. Transactional changes need to stay updated on the latest developments, especially when they focus on specific organizational issues like the latest vaccines and the state of quantum computer development (Bhattacharyya 2020). In contrast, transformation changes are more holistic and require effective use of change strategies, pacing with environmental and technological trends such as quantum computer development (Bhattacharyya 2020).

Lewin's change management model and Kolter's model of change, both popular prescriptive models of organizational change, could benefit by using quantum algorithms as a framework (Bhattacharyya 2020). Additionally, there are different stages that could be monitored by future quantum computers, such as the urgency for change, building teams for change, constructing and communicating team vision, and equally empowering the creation of short-term goals and long-term persistency (Bhattacharyya 2020). The problem is that this model is time-consuming and would be considered a luxury in the current pandemic situation. Quantum computing, however, could more easily handle the situation due to the way it handles vast amounts of simultaneous data (Bhattacharyya 2020). Addressing the current COVID-19 pandemic is a complicated organizational change issue, requiring organizational restructuring and reengineering. Such future situations could be handled much more quickly and efficiently with the introduction of quantum computing. However, current data could be used to pilot methods and algorithms for quantum computers before we experience another pandemic (Bhattacharyya 2020).

Some companies made a true effort during the pandemic to address change management. For example, many companies repurposed their production to address personal protective equipment shortages; insurance companies in the Al Kahtani (2020) study put change management at the heart of everything they did and ensured no business disruption, which in turn ensured sustainability (Al Kahtani 2020). The study concluded that a positive relationship existed between change management practices and organizational culture; the hypothesis that organizational culture mediates the relationship between change management practices and organizational success was supported (Al Kahtani 2020).

8. Quantum Computers, Pandemics, and Change Management Developments

Until now we have been studying change management through semantics and through academic studies on pandemics or quantum computers. Now we are going to look at the pandemic in conjunction with the advent of future quantum computers. The Hawthorn effect stipulates that individuals behave differently when observed. In a sense, this is change management or the analysis of change and the effect of an external stimulus like a vaccine. Even after the pandemic, vaccines were developed and distributed; everyone had to wear a mask in public places and for those unvaccinated, temperatures were regularly taken—individuals were being observed very closely, which was a direct adaption to change. This is reminiscent of Winston Smith in George Orwell's *1984*. Future studies will tell how this constant electronic thermal eye (or Future quantum computer thermal camera) affects future generations of workers even though the reason for thermal eye is altruistic, since it tells the temperature of employees who might carry infection.

The constant invasiveness of technology will only increase with the advent of a quantum internet (QI) which would require quantum communication between various remote nodes (Singh et al. 2021, 1). The change management adaption to QI in the future will help with addressing the challenge of pandemics. The future holds in store several developments in quantum channels guarded by quantum cryptographic protocols, and these protocols will include change management and the planned reaction to pandemics (Singh et al. 2021). In this futuristic quantum computer world of pandemics and change management, such networks would rely on quantum bits (qubits) that have properties of superposition, entanglement, tunneling, annealing and teleportation, consequently providing an edge to quantum networks over traditional networks (Singh et al. 2021). Future technology could transmit qubits over long distances, currently a formidable task, which is why there is currently extensive research on satellite-based quantum communication. Such communication could provide instantaneously shared information on a global scale regarding pandemic data (Singh et al. 2021). It is clear that "the three-qubit space consisting of a superconducting qubit, an oscillator, and an atomic qubit, leading to the potentials of tailoring two-qubit entangled state" will most likely help with pandemics in a change management framework (Yu et al. 2017, 2).

9. Addressing the Potential for Change Management and Quantum Computer Errors

To address the change management problem of errors, which already exists in modern computers in the form of error-correcting code (ECC), researchers have studied different scenarios. One of these solutions is the probabilities of a situation "associated with engineering fast, programmable interactions between spin qubits separated by micrometer-scale distances" (Rosenfeld et al. 2021, 2061). The science of probabilities, in conjunction with the pandemic and change management, could offer up a study of *color centers* such as the diamond nitrogen-vacancy (NV) center are promising contenders as robust qubits, owing to their long coherence times at room temperature" (Rosenfeld et al. 2021, 2061). If nitrogen-vacancy becomes a breakthrough, it could be the center of a new change management policy to find solutions to future pandemics. In recent developments, IonQ achieved the trapped ion quantum computation of 160-bit storage qubits, which will offer more data storage for change management protocols and quantum computer data (Li and Cai 2021). In conjunction with this, for *diamond spin systems*, some techniques can be used to improve scaling of quantum networks relying on phosphorus in silicon 19, quantum dots; this will also be a useful technology to approach future pandemics in an environment of change management (Waldherr et al. 2014).

A succinct explanation of what an *eigenvalue* represents is a multi-part and will eventually become ubiquitous in a change management project involving pandemics. First, an eigenvalue is explained by the fact that "|x> represents the state of the particle in which we know with certainty to find the particle at position x" and since change management pandemic projects are scientific in nature, solving for x will be the goal (Casati 2021a, 78). In this case, the x to solve for the pandemic change management project will be in a "Hilbert space, x" (Casati 2021a, 108). Hilbert space is a limited space allowing for classical calculus, which can be applied to a change management pandemic project. The Hilbert space x is in "the eigenstate[s] of position," which can also be applied in a change management project (Casati 2021a, 108). An Eigenstate can also be described strictly in terms of energy and a "Hamiltonian is the sum of potential and kinetic energy for the particles in a system," which can directly apply to studying a pandemic (Casati 2020a, 108).

Conjunctly, an *Ansätze* architecture search (AAS) algorithm was proposed to study quantum computers, which can in turn help a change management pandemic project (Li et al. 2020, 2). Ansätze is related to heuristics, the science of random events, directly correlated to change management projects related to the pandemic (Casati 2020). Casati (2021b) determined that the properties of atoms and molecules can be determined by solving the Schrodinger equation, which can also be used for the pandemic in the form of a change management project. Likewise, in the field of quantum computational chemistry (QCC) (i.e., quantum chemistry run on quantum computers) a change management project can be drawn towards addressing a pandemic (Poirier and Jerke 2021). QCC will be useful during pandemics to track change management. This will advance the science of quantum computers, which will in turn advance knowledge on pandemics and change management variants. The ground state is calculated by calculating the sum of two contributions (Kirby et al. 2021). The "first contribution comes from a non-contextual approximation to the Hamiltonian and is computed classically" (Kirby et al. 2021, 1). The "second contribution is obtained by using the variational quantum *eigensolver* (VQE) technique to compute a contextual correction on a quantum processor" (Kirby et al. 2021, 1).

10. Change Management Data during a Pandemic for Future Quantum Computers

In a manuscript by Ludvigon (2021), the data in figure 4 shows that the number of telehealth encounters increased from 150,000 in 2009 to 1,074,000 in 2018. This is an exponential increase which shows a societal shift occurring from discomfort with technology in the past to the current population which trusts computers more. The current awareness of antivirus, antispyware, firewalls, intrusion detection systems, and intrusion prevention systems is due to the increase of attacks on personal information (Casati et al. 2018). Quantum computers, however, will hopefully be less prone to infections and increase fluidity in change management projects.

Quantum computer research is going to benefit and change management projects that grow from the use and overuse of computers during the pandemic. In a study by Panaitescu and Renea (2020), connectivity and the use of internet services and integration of digital technology and digital public services were analyzed, and it was abundantly clear that the weighted index was high for industrialized counties but much lower for underdeveloped economies in Eastern Europe (Panaitescu and Renea 2020). This weighted index suggests that change management pandemic-centric projects for less industrialized countries are less accessible. This disparity shows that pandemics affect world economies in different ways, which means their patients are also treated with less effectiveness and relentlessness than western economies.

Quantum computers will have to develop their own change management projects, but telecommunication software development has provided significant improvements during the pandemic. In a study by Khan et al. (2020), it was clear that *Microsoft Teams*, a software for teleconferencing was used in most scenarios, Blackboard *Collaborate*, and *Moodle* were the top three in use for virtual classes, while Zoom and Google Classrooms were tied for fourth place. However, the frequency of use and cost of virtual meeting programs show different percentages depending on their application. These virtual meeting and collaboration programs saved the global economy during the pandemic and future programs designed for quantum computers will most likely outperform all of them in this intellectual property space.

Change management has been a great tool for companies recently, and they have leveraged this instrument in surveying their employees. The conclusion reached in such a survey by Irimiás and Mitev (2020) was that change management was an integral part of the corporate culture during the pandemic and that technology such as quantum computers would prevail in the future. It was also argued that strategic change, innovative opportunities, and more capability were higher than average using a Likert scale yet only reached a high of three out of five points. Unsurprisingly moderate results were recorded by Hadi and Irbah Athallah (2021) with gamification learning which was trialed during the pandemic. Future quantum computers will be able to process this data using the methodologies optimized for the new computing platform.

11. Statistics Related to the Pandemic

Future analysis of pandemics would benefit from more advanced computing such as quantum computers, which do not use traditional central processing units; however, it is not clear how quantum computers would be used in the future (Alexeev et al. 2021). It is extremely challenging to focus the development of qubit technologies at the component level to work on pandemics using change management (Alexeev et al. 2021). The review of the literature on quantum computing suggests the practical interest in quantum computing arose from the discovery that there are certain computational problems, such as number factoring that can be solved more efficiently on a quantum computer than on a classical computer (Alexeev et al. 2021). Number factoring, which could be utilized in a change management project for pandemics, is used in Shor's algorithm, recently presented at the MBAA conference (Casati 2021b).

The mathematical harmony of quantum computing is not the only advantage to a specifically pandemic-focused change management project. The quantitative aspect of the pandemic often overshadows the human element. As if the Facebook whistleblower Frances Haugen's opinion was self-prophesying (that fixing negativity-driven algorithms would erase our flawed humanity). While working on a pandemic-focused change management project, the advantage of a quantum computer is that it does not operate at extremely inefficient heat dissipation of 10^{10}

kT per bit copied (Casati 2021b). Instead, a quantum computer operates at an efficiency level close to the DNA heat dissipation of 100 kT per bit copied, which could be used in a change management project focused on a pandemic (Casati 2020). There is also an alternative research and development stage computing device to quantum computers, which is DNA computing (Casati, 2020). DNA is an acronym which stands for deoxyribonucleic acid. DNA is made of four building blocks which are adenine, cytosine, guanine, and thymine. In 1994, Leonard Adleman thought of using these four building blocks as a computer. Using DNA as a computer is faster, it is small to store information, and it has low heat dissipation as described above. In this case, the state vector $|\Psi>$, also called a ket and its matching $<\Psi|$ called a bra are also an integral part of DNA computing (Casati, 2021a, p. 80). $|\Psi>$ is equal to $a|1> + b|0>$. The Dirac notation of $|1>$ and $|0>$ represent two vectors (Casati 2021a, 80). Furthermore, the "superposition of $|0>$ and $|1>$ or the existence in both states" could be illustrated in four different ways (Casati 2021a, 80) either 00, 01, 10, or 11. Since there are four different notations for the pairs of zeros and ones, they could be mapped onto the following four nucleotide bases: adenine, cytosine, guanine, and thymine in DNA to then be programmed into a DNA based Quantum Computer.

The possible combinations for an experiment vary and different researchers have mapped different combinations of DNA building blocks to different combinations of zeros and ones. An example of this, among many others, could be illustrated as follows:

00 could be mapped as adenine

01 could be mapped as cytosine

10 could be mapped as guanine

11 could be mapped as thymine

According to Casati (2019), artificial intelligence will soon play a greater role in quantum computing. Quantum computers have states of superposition and entanglement. Superposition is the coexistence of different microstate values of the same particle at the same time (both 1 and 0), so the quantum computer can simultaneously evaluate microstate values of 10, 01, 11, and 00 (Casati 2021b). Entanglement means there is a strong microstate correlation between otherwise spatially separated particles (Casati 2021a). There is evidence that entangled particles behave as a single entitle despite their spatial separation. According to Casati (2021b), two other concepts that distinguish classical computers from quantum computers are tunneling—the ability to go through multiple layers of data—and annealing—which is finding the overall minimum of value microstates (e.g., 10, 01, 11, and 00).

The importance of this concept is that a DNA/quantum computer could take advantage of this interface between DNA mapping and a binary system, benefitting research on future pandemics from this type of living computer (Casati and Thakkar 2018). Algorithms could be written to interface between pandemics like COVID-19 DNA and a DNA computer. Mohamad et al. (2009), Saaid (2009), and others have published papers on similar techniques for DNA computing.

On a similar topic, coulomb blockades result in devices with transistor-like characteristics, which further advance the possibility of an actual functional quantum computer that could help with a pandemic-focused change management project (Casati 2021a). Moreover, it can be posited that Shor's algorithm for factoring integers is an example of where a quantum computer outperforms classical computers focused on a potential change management project related to a future pandemic (Casati 2021a).

When conducting any type of experiment like DNA computing, it is important to consider the *internal validity instrumentation threats* and the *external validity threats* to the equation models presented in this change management model (Casati 2012). The predictability, reliability, reproducibility, validity of the DNA building blocks presented above are to the best of the author's knowledge at an acceptable level. It is equally important that all internal validity and external validity threats have been considered carefully.

A DNA computer model using a Gaussian curve model, as described earlier in this chapter, illustrates a "shaded area below the curve will represent the total number of cases" during a pandemic (Jozaghi 2020). Yamada et al. (2021) explained the state of the pandemic world we all live in extremely well, recounting how over one year ago, a new pandemic emerged, not only affected the healthcare sector, but also the economy and the public's morale. In the retelling of this story, Yamada et al. (2021) stated in the epilogue that authorities used draconian measures to keep the pandemic from going viral; in some cases, all social contacts were banned, businesses and schools were closed, threats of arrest for those exiting their homes who had been diagnosed as being COVID positive, and all these measures occurring in a very short period (educational, transactional, and professional forums almost all went online). Although online teaching and learning required changes in education management (Suman et al. 2020), societies cried tyranny due to the egregiousness and often conflicting nature of science versus politics associated with these new regulations.

12. Summary

During the pandemic, various computer communication programs and services were used for global communications purposes. While these programs were effectively used on conventional computers, it will eventually be possible to run pandemic algorithms and change management problems on quantum computational chemistry devices assisted by DNA computers to ensure businesses and supply chains are not disrupted and remain reliable and sustainable. DNA computers have the distinct advantage of being *living* organisms and *could theoretically build* quantum gate computers. In terms of the current pandemic, restructuring and reengineering will become ubiquitous. The businesses which adapted well during the pandemic will continue to improve their processes while those who were less fortunate by the nature of the business or inability to rapidly adapt to the changing environment, will need to focus and be conscious of their core organizational structure, culture, and change management issues.

The accidents and essence of the pandemic depend on which way the problem is analyzed, which begs the question of how future quantum computers will approach the problem. If the future quantum computers approach the problem of the pandemic more through policies rather than through corporate policies there might be some backlash or resistance to change. A wise approach is through karma or action, rather than substance. Therefore, political agendas need to be abandoned when addressing societal needs during a pandemic. The needs of any political party should not replace the needs of all parties, which are collectively the needs of the entire population. Political misuse of information, disinformation, fear-mongering, woke movement backlashes, and policies that conflict with scientific data for political leverage must be avoided at all costs. Trust is paramount to public acceptance of vaccines and the freedom to choose must replace mandates that reflect overarching control rather than encouragement to participate for the benefit of the public. Shaming, demonizing, Orwellian, and dystopic rhetoric and other negative communication and representation by media outlets need to be called out for their abuses so the public trust in their leaders is maintained throughout periods of significant social strife, whether caused by a pandemic, social unrest, war, or other environmental disasters.

Without the ability to quickly analyze a broad spectrum of data, change management projects designed to address a pandemic, especially involving quantum computers, will most likely fail, maybe due to excessive change or lack of communication. The world during the pandemic has lost its way and focused more on profits and political leveraging of events. The profits and political capitalization are directly correlated to the pandemic and financially commensurate with the fear inspired by media outlets that proposed doomsday scenarios and attributed even marginally associated fatalities with the pandemic.

The quantum gate computer has not yet been proven to function on an industrial scale unlike the adiabatic quantum computer, yet advances in quantum computing are ongoing and future versions of quantum computers may rely on technology as yet undeveloped. Concurrent to advances in quantum computing, the biological sciences have made significant strides in only the past few years due in large part to the reaction to the pandemic, so it is only natural to posit that change management will play a greater role in business and the biological sciences in the years ahead. As the pandemic is coming under control and we are striving to prevent yet another global epidemic, it will be important to take change management under serious consideration and wisely choose to increase the priority in developing the technology to achieve quantum computing, especially as a change management tool for a global disaster such as a pandemic.

Change management project models will continue to evolve as a result of advances in technology and the convergence of physical and social environmental events and quantum computer development. The barriers between diametrically separate industries are bound to fall since every industry is destined to depend on the collection and processing of accurate data.

References

Alexeev, Y., Bacon, D., Brown, K. R., Calderbank, R., Carr, L. D., Chong, F. T., DeMarco, B., Englund, D., Farhi, E., Fefferman, B., Gorshkov, A. V., Houck, A., Kim, J., Kimmel, S., Lange, M. Lloyd, S., Lukin, M. D., Maslov, D., Maunz, P., . . . Thompson, J. 2021. "Quantum computer systems for scientific discovery." *PRX Quantum*, *2* (1), https://doi.org/10.1103/PRXQuantum.2.017001

Al Kahtani, M. 2020. "The change management strategy in the private sector insurance companies after COVID-19." *Journal of Research in Administrative Sciences* (ISSN: 2664-2433), *9* (1), 12–18. https://jraspublications.org/index.php/jras/article/download/42/56

Archibong, U., and Ibrahim, U. A. 2021. "Assessing the impact of change management on employee performance: Evidence from Nile University of Nigeria." *International Journal of Research in Business and Social Science* (2147-4478), 10 (4): 525–534. https://doi.org/10.20525/ijrbs.v10i4.1246

Barrow, J., M., Annamaraju, P., and Toney-Butler, T., J. 2017. *Change Management*. StatPearls Publishing.

Bhattacharyya, D. K. 2020. "Normative change management model in COVID-19 pandemic." *Journal of Research in Administrative Sciences* (ISSN: 2664-2433), 9(1): 19–21. https://doi.org/10.47609/JRAS2020v9i1p3

Casati, N. M. 2021a. "Use of quantum computers in understanding cultures and global business successes." In *Culture in Global*

Businesses: Addressing National and Organizational Challenges, edited by B. S. Thakkar, 77–103. Palgrave Macmillan.

Casati, N. M. 2021b. "Using Shor's algorithm for integer factorization in quantum

computers: An approach to equality" (March 24–26) (Conference presentation) MBAA 2021 Conference, Chicago, IL, United States. MBAA 2021 Conference, Chicago, IL, United States. https://mbaainternational.org/wp-content/uploads/2022/01/MBAA-Conference-

Schedule-2021_FINAL-TO-POST.pdf

Casati, N. M. 2020. "Current and future global challenges in management and leadership: Finance and quantum computing." In *Paradigm Shift in Management Philosophy: Future Challenges in Global Organizations,* edited by B. S. Thakkar, 103–131. Palgrave Macmillan.

Casati, N. M. 2019. Investigation of the Role of Artificial Intelligence in the Future of Leadership (March 27–29) (Conference presentation). MBAA 2019 Conference, Chicago, IL, United States. https://mbaainternational.org/wp-content/uploads/2019/04/MBAA-Program-2019-FINAL-AFTER-CONF.pdf

Casati, N. M., Kesavabhotla, K., and Cybulski, G. R. 2018. "Future of leadership in healthcare business: A global perspective." In *The Future of Leadership: Addressing Complex Global Issues,* edited by B. S. Thakkar, 197–228. Palgrave Macmillan.

Casati, N. M., and Thakkar, B. S. 2018. "Technology Growth and Businesses in Global

Markets" (April 18–20) (Conference presentation) MBAA 2018 Conference, Chicago, IL, United States.

https://mbaainternational.org/wp-content/uploads/2018/05/MBAA-Program-2018-Whole-Post-Conference.pdf

Casati, F. 1992. *Le Thermometre de Lyon*. Lyon, FR: Edition

Lyonnaise d'Art et d'Histoire.

CBInsights. 2021. *What is quantum computing? Definition, industry trends, and benefits explained*. https://www.cbinsights.com/research/report/quantum-computing/

Dubé, M., Kaba, A., Cronin, T., Barnes, S., Fuselli, T., and Grant, V. 2020. "COVID-19 pandemic preparation: Using simulation for systems-based learning to prepare the largest healthcare workforce and system in Canada." *Advances in Simulation, 5* (22): 1–12. https://doi.org/10.1186/s41077-020-00138-w

Edmunds, C. L. 2021. Error Characterisation and Reduction in Trapped Ion Quantum

Computers—One Woman's Guide to the Ion-ing (Doctoral dissertation, The University of Sydney). https://ses.library.usyd.edu.au/bitstream/handle/2123/25668/edmunds_cl_thesis.pdf?sequence=1&isAllowed=y

Gill, R. 2002. Change management--or change leadership? *Journal of Change Management*, 3 (4), 307–318. https://doi.org/10.1080/714023845

Khan, S., Rabbani, R. M., Thalassinos, I. E., and Atif, M. 2020. "Corona virus pandemic paving ways to next generation of learning and teaching: Futuristic cloud-based educational model." *SSRN* (August 8). https://dx.doi.org/10.2139/ssrn.3669832

Kirby, W. M., Tranter, A., and Love, P. J. 2021. "Contextual subspace variational quantum Eigensolver." *Quantum, 5:* 456. https://doi.org/10.22331/q-2021-05-14-456

Hadi, M. S., and irbah Athallah, N. I. 2021. "Gamification's Effectiveness in Online English Teaching in the Pandemic Era." *Jurnal Studi Guru Dan Pembelajaran, 4* (2): 282–286. https://e-journal.my.id/jsgp/article/view/590

Hayes, J. 2018. *The Theory and Practice of Change Management,* 5th ed. Palgrave.

Hoek, R. V. 2020. "Responding to COVID-19 supply chain risks—Insights from supply chain change management, total cost of ownership and supplier segmentation theory." *Logistics,* 4 (4) (September 23): https://doi.org/10.3390/logistics4040023

Irimiás, A., and Mitev, A. 2020. "Change management, digital maturity, and green development: Are successful firms leveraging on sustainability?" *Sustainability,* 12 (10) (May 14): 4019. https://doi.org/10.3390/su12104019

Jozaghi, Y. 2020. "Coronavirus disease 2019—the principles of the curve, explained simply." *Head & Neck,* 42 (7): 1539–1542. https://doi.org/10.1002/hed.26289

Kak, S. 2019. "A quantum computing future is unlikely, due to random hardware errors" (December 3). The Conversation. https://theconversation.com/a-quantum-computing-future-is-unlikely-due-to-random-hardware-errors-126503

Lauer, T. 2010. *Change Management: Fundamentals and Success Factors.* Springer.

Lewin, K. 1997. *Resolving Social Conflicts and Field Theory in Social Science.* American Psychological Association. https://doi.org/10.1037/10269-000

Li, K., and Cai, Qy. 2021. "Practical security of RSA against NTC-Architecture quantum computing attacks." *International Journal of Theoretical Physics*, 60 (June 19): 2733–2744. https://doi. org/10.1007/s10773-021-04789-x

Li, L., Fan, M., Coram, M., Riley, P., and Leichenauer, S. 2020. "Quantum optimization with a novel Gibbs objective function and ansatz architecture search." *Physical Review Research*, 2 (April 24), 023074. https://doi.org/10.1103/PhysRevResearch.2.023074

Ludvigson, T. 2021. *Leveraging Virtual Technology to Support the Operational Capability of the Department of Veterans Affairs amidst a Global Pandemic* (Seminar paper presented to graduate faculty at UW Platteville). Platteville, WI. http://digital.library. wisc.edu/1793/82136

Mohamad, M.S., Omatu, S., Deris, S., Misman, M. F., and Yoshioka, M. 2009. "A multi-objective strategy in genetic algorithms for gene selection of gene expression data." *Artificial Life and Robotics* 13 (March 8): 410–413. https://doi.org/10.1007/s10015-008-0533-5

Panaitescu, M., and Renea, P. 2020. "Change management in tourism in the context of the COVID 19 pandemic." *Univ. Agric. Sci. Vet. Med. Iasi*, *74*, 156–161. https://pesquisa.bvsalud.org/ global-literature-on-novel-coronavirus-2019-ncov/resource/pt/ covidwho-995543?lang=en

Poirier, B., and Jerke, J. 2021. *Full-Dimensional Schrodinger Wavefunction Calculations Using Tensors and Quantum Computers: The Cartesian Component-Separated Approach* (May 8). Cornell University. https://arxiv.org/pdf/2105.03787.pdf

Roşca, V. I. 2020. "Implications of Lewin's field theory on social change." In *Proceedings of the International Conference on Business Excellence,* 14 (1) (July 26): 617–625. Sciendo. https:// doi.org/10.2478/picbe-2020-0058

Rosenfeld, E., Riedinger, R., Gieseler, J., Schuetz, M., and Lukin, M. D. 2021. "Efficient entanglement of spin qubits mediated by a hot mechanical oscillator." *Physical Review Letters*, 126 (25). https:// doi.org/10.1103/PhysRevLett.126.250505

Saaid, M. F. M. 2009. *Clustering Techniques for DNA Computing Readout Method Based on Real-Time Polymerase Chain Reaction* (Master's thesis, Universiti Teknologi Malaysia). http://eprints.utm.my/id/ eprint/18194/1/MuhammadFaizMohamedSaaidMFKE2009.pdf

Shuman, V., Sander, D., and Scherer, K. R. 2013. Levels of valence. *Frontiers in Psychology*, 4 (May 13): 261. https://doi.org/10.3389/ fpsyg.2013.00261

Singh, A., Dev, K., Siljak, H., Joshi, H. D., and Magarini, M. 2021. "Quantum internet-applications, functionalities, enabling technologies, challenges, and research directions." *Cornell University* (June 1). Retrieved October 10, 2021. https://arxiv. org/pdf/2101.04427.pdf

Sridhar, M. K., and Nagendra, H. R. 2018. *Consciousness in Indian Philosophy and Modern Physics* (September 25–29) (Paper). National Workshop on Writing Indian Philosophy in Modern Perspective, Sanchi University of Buddhist-Indic Studies, Academic Campus, Barla (Raisen).https://library.sanchiuniv.edu. in/indian-philosophy-conf-proceeding/

Suman, P., Srivastava, R., and Saxena, A. 2020. "Online teaching and learning in management education during pandemic: Student perspective." *Psychology and Education Journal*, 57 (9): 5177– 5185. http://psychologyandeducation.net/pae/index.php/pae/ article/view/2059

Tran, A., Sudre, B., Paz, S., Rossi, M., Desbrosse, A., Chevalier, V., and Semenza, J. C. 2014. "Environmental predictors of West Nile fever risk in Europe." *International Journal of Health Geographics*, 13 (1) (July 1), 1–11. https://doi.org/10.1186/1476-072X-13-26

United States Government Accountability Office (US GAO). 2021. *Operation Warp Speed: Accelerated COVID-19 Vaccine Development Status and Efforts to Address Manufacturing Challenges* (February). https://www.gao.gov/assets/720/712410.pdf

Vermeiren, F. 2021. "Whitehead and the immanence of extension." *Process Studies*, 50 (2): 201–221. https://www.jstor.org/stable/10.5406/processstudies.50.2.0201

Waldherr, G., Wang, Y., Zaiser, S., Jamali, M., Schulte-Herbrüggen, T., Abe, H., and Wrachtrup, J. 2014. "Quantum error correction in a solid-state hybrid spin register." *Nature*, 506 (February 12): 204–207. https://doi.org/10.1038/nature12919

Wang, Z., Marcellina, E., Hamilton, A. R., Cullen, J. H., Rogge, S., Salfi, J., and Culcer, D. 2021. "Optimal operation points for ultrafast, highly coherent Ge hole spin-orbit qubits." *Quantum Information*, 7 (54) (April 1): 1–8. https://doi.org/10.1038/s41534-021-00386-2

Xu, J. Ye, J. 2020. "Perspectives on supercomputing and artificial intelligence applications in drug discovery." *Supercomputing Frontiers and Innovations*, 7 (3). https://doi.org/10.14529/jsfi200302

Yamada, Y., Ćepulić, D. B., Coll-Martín, T., Debove, S., Gautreau, G., Han, H., and Lieberoth, A. 2021. "COVIDiSTRESS global survey dataset on psychological and behavioural consequences of the COVID-19 outbreak." *Scientific Data*, 8 (3) (January 4): 1–23. https://doi.org/10.1038/s41597-020-00784-9

Yu, D., Kwek, L. C., Amico, L., and Dumke, R. 2017. "Superconducting qubit-resonator-atom hybrid system." *Quantum Science and Technology*, 2 (3) (July 28). https://doi.org/10.1088/2058-9565/aa7c50

CHAPTER 10

A Journalist's Perspective: COVID-19 and How It Upended the World

by Mayank Chhaya

Abstract

Viruses have existed for millions of years as we understand them now, according to a study by scientists at Boston College. To those born in the latter half of the twentieth century and early twenty-first century, it is only the rise of the COVID-19 or Coronavirus disease 2019 that has brought about an awareness of what viruses are and the devastation they can cause. The last comparable pandemic was the influenza pandemic of 1918–1919 that killed some 50 million people globally. Compare that with a little over 4.9 million deaths and 245 million total cases created by the COVID-19 as of the end of October 2021, and it begins to tell a story of extraordinary advances in vaccine development and distribution over the last century.

Notwithstanding, the COVID-19 pandemic has upended the way the world functions, right from global health systems to supply chains and from jobs to societal balance. This chapter offers a broad journalistic perspective on how life has been fundamentally altered in the time of the pandemic on every known yardstick.

Keywords: Viruses, COVID-19, pandemic, global health systems

A Journalist's Perspective

Viruses have existed for between 15 and 30 million years as we understand them now, according to a study by scientists at Boston College. However, they were discovered barely 130 years in 1892 when Dmitry Iosifovich Ivanovsky, a Russian microbiologist, during his study of mosaic disease in tobacco, chanced upon it. He was the one who first detailed many characteristics of the organisms that were christened virus six years later by a Dutch botanist named M. W. Beijerinck.

It is believed that Ivanovsky may not have fully understood the importance of his discovery. It was Beijerinck whose work gave it the discipline that gradually went on to become the science of virology it has now become.

However, the study of ancient viruses is of recent vintage with the emergence of genome sequencing and high-volume data analysis which has allowed scientists to look tens of millions of years into the past. The Boston College study team was led by professor of biology Welkin Johnson which found the global spread of an ancient group of retroviruses dating back between 15 and 30 million years. The retroviruses affected about 28 of 50 modern mammals' ancestors, according to this study.

It is not readily realized by people that viruses have existed as long as there has been life on earth. Professor Johnson has been quoted by an official Boston University announcement as saying, "Viruses have been with us for billions of years and exist everywhere that life is found. They therefore have a significant impact on the ecology and evolution of all organisms, from bacteria to humans. Unfortunately, viruses do not leave fossils behind, meaning we know very little about how they originate and evolve."

The announcement dated September 6, 2021, said, "Retroviruses are abundant in nature and include human immunodeficiency viruses [HIV-1 and -2] and human T-cell leukemia viruses. The scientists' findings on a specific group of these viruses called ERV-Fc, published in the journal eLife, show that they affected a wide range of hosts, including species as diverse as carnivores, rodents, and primates.

"The distribution of ERV-Fc among these ancient mammals suggests the viruses spread to every continent except Antarctica and Australia, and that they jumped from one species to another more than 20 times.

As the world struggles with the COVID-19, short for Coronavirus 2019, and its variants such as delta, which originated in India in December 2020 and mu, which was first identified in Colombia in January 2021, there appears to be a general apprehension among communities across the world that the human race will have to learn to live with mutations. According to the World Health Organization (WHO), mu is the fifth variant of the virus which has fundamentally altered the way societies now function.

Perhaps unlike any viruses before, the COVID-19 has had such a sweeping political consequence in a country like the United States that oftentimes the politics of the virus is far more predominant in public discourse than the science of the virus. For some bizarre reasons, acknowledging the seriousness of the virus and trying to address it at various levels, such as wearing masks and getting vaccinated, has become a deeply divisive issue in America with those adhering to the right of center or the extreme right of center political ideologies choosing to condemn them in the vilest terms.

In some quarters not wearing masks and not getting vaccinated have become signs of machismo among those who swear blind allegiance to perhaps the most absurdly irresponsible assertions that former Pres. Donald Trump made about the pandemic early on. For instance, on April 23, 2020, the president of the world's most scientifically advanced nation advised citizens from the White House press room to inject bleach into their bodies to fight the virus. Even by his generally lunatic standards, this was a dangerously irresponsible assertion.

Sample this verbatim stream of consciousness coming from Trump that horrified the world. "A question that probably some of you are thinking of if you're totally into that world. So, supposing we hit the body with a tremendous—whether it's ultraviolet or just very powerful light—and I think you said that that hasn't been checked, but you're going to test it. And then I said, supposing you brought the light inside the body, which you can do either through the skin or in some other way, and I think you said you're going to test that, too. It sounds interesting. And then I see the disinfectant, where it knocks it out in a minute. One minute. And is there a way we can do something like that, by injection inside or almost a cleaning. Because you see it gets in the lungs, and it does a tremendous number on the lungs. So it would be interesting to check that."

The idea that you could drink bleach in a manner of speaking or inject sunlight to fight the virus was so insane by any measure that it should have been rejected across the political spectrum. However, there was a significant number of people who found it worthwhile. Political tribalism devouring serious medical science was on a deeply embarrassing display throughout Trump's one year of dealing with the pandemic. What was particularly galling was that while he was dishing out these witch-doctor cures to his unsuspecting and ignorant camp followers, he himself was receiving some of the most expensive medical treatment from his own COVID-19 infection. He was eventually reported to have got himself vaccinated as well even while ridiculing the efficacy of vaccines for the consumption of his followers.

Trump's departure from the White House did not mean that the number of the profoundly ignorant populace of supporters he created was reduced. In fact, political opposition to the incoming president Joe Biden among his supporters exacerbated and assumed the role of a kind of revolt by many who continued to reject the COVID vaccine purely on the grounds of politics. So sharpened the divide became that one could predict with a fair amount of certainty that those who rejected the virus as a problem and therefore rejected its vaccines were also the ones who rejected Biden as a legitimate president swayed by Trump's manifestly absurd claims about the *stolen election.*

At least in the US context, the virus did not just remain a problem of virology and public health but became a disturbingly partisan political issue with a direct bearing on the future of the country. Shock jocks and rabidly right-wing television talking heads relentlessly poisoned the public mind with vicious conspiracy theories about the virus as a result of which across middle and southern America, traditionally known to be the bastion of conservative Republic politics and ideology, millions rejected both masks and vaccination. The result of this willful disregard of common sense and science led to the country topping 700,000 deaths. It was a staggering number considering that vaccines started becoming widely available soon after President Biden take over as his administration benefited partly from the war-footing vaccine research and production under Trump in the latter half of his last year in 2020.

What was troubling about a spike in deaths from July 2021 in the aftermath of the emergence of the delta variant was that a majority of these deaths was occurring among the unvaccinated, most of whom were in the south egged on by anti-vaxxer conspiracists who peddled theories such as vaccines being a Trojan horse to embed electronic chips in people to track them or that it magnetized the human body. Belief in such ludicrous claims significantly explained the fact that between July 2021 and September 2021, deaths due to the virus increased nearly tenfold from 1,525 per week to 14,220 in a particular week in September, according to Johns Hopkins University's data.

The cruel irony in the US was that while there was a glut in the vaccine supply, even as the rest of the world scrambled to get some, millions of Americans refused them. The clearest fallout of that rejection was that between June 16, 2021, and September 29, 2021, 95,232 people died in 105 days with a majority being unvaccinated.

The COVID pandemic became America's deadliest pandemic in history, surpassing the influenza pandemic of 1918–1919 that killed some 675,000 people. The fact that over a century of revolutionary advances in not just vaccine development but vaccine manufacturing capacity, delivery, and communications tools for public messaging about the pandemic did not help America save those lost. A great deal of that had to do with the politics of the pandemic rather than the science of it.

Media reporting and scholarly discourse about the COVID pandemic frequently invoked the flu pandemic of 1918–19 because it was for the first time in a century that the world was hit by a pandemic matching in scale and potential lethality. The flu pandemic infected about a third of the world population then of some 1.8 billion people or about 500 million people. It killed some 50 million people globally with the US number totaling about 675,000. It is important to remember that the 1918 flu deaths came in the midst of a complete absence of any vaccine. As pointed out by U.S. Centers for Disease Control (CDC), "With no vaccine to protect against influenza infection and no antibiotics to treat secondary bacterial infections that can be associated with influenza infections, control efforts worldwide were limited to non-pharmaceutical interventions such as isolation, quarantine, good personal hygiene, use of disinfectants, and limitations of public gatherings, which were applied unevenly."

The flu pandemic grotesquely highlighted the health and economic inequities that ruled the world, a significant portion of which was still under the control of British imperial rule. India, often called the Jewel in the British Crown because of its many riches, was the worst hit by the flu that killed between 17 and 18 million people, which was about six percent of its total population. More women and children, whose immunities were devastated by malnourishment and starvation, died due to the flu than men.

So indiscriminate and unsparing was the flu's spread in India that even Mohandas Gandhi did not escape it. He along with his fellow inmates at his ashram in the city of Ahmedabad in Gujarat remained sick for several days. For Gandhi, it was his first protracted illness.

In his much-regarded memoir *A Life Misspent*, Suryakant Tripathi, one of Hindi literature's most heralded poets who wrote under the name Nirala, recalled the flu's devastating effects in some detail. "I travelled to the riverbank in Dalmau and waited," he wrote, "the Ganga was swollen with dead bodies. At my in-laws' house, I learned that my wife had passed away." Nirala lost many others in his family and mentioned that there was not enough wood to cremate them.

"This was the strangest time in my life," he recalled. "My family disappeared in the blink of an eye. All our sharecroppers and laborers died, the four who worked for my cousin, as well as the two who worked for me. My cousin's eldest son was fifteen years old, my young daughter a year old. In whichever direction I turned, I saw darkness." These deaths were not just a coincidence of personal tragedies visited upon the poet, they were connected. "The newspapers had informed us about the ravages of the epidemic," Nirala wrote.

The flu pandemic occurred in the pre-antibiotic and for a large swath of the world, pre-independence era. The period around 1918 was considered the high noon of the British Empire which really could not care less about what the flu pandemic did to the native populations. The deaths of some 18 million Indians due to the flu pandemic did not appear to have dented Britain's grip over the colonized world much since it took another three decades for its colonies to become free.

In sheer statistical terms, the 1918 flu pandemic and the COVID-19 pandemic are not comparable. Take for instance, the death to infections ratio in 1918-1919. Of the 500 million people who were infected by the flu virus in 1918-1919, 50 million or 10 percent died. In contrast as of October 1, 2021, of the little over 234 million cases of the COVID 19 infection globally a little over 4.7 million people died or about two percent. That relatively low number could be attributed to several factors, including considerably to the rapid vaccine development and distribution as well as the overall improvement in public health infrastructure compared to a century ago.

The flu pandemic ravaged populations under oppressive colonization where the colonizing power, namely Britain was criminally apathetic to the people it subjugated. Add to that the fact that it followed in the immediate aftermath of World War I which had devastated Europe, the home to all the traditional colonizers such as France,

Britain, Portugal, and the Dutch. Not that there is any reason to believe that in the absence of the war Britain would have found it within its collective conscience to handle it more humanely.

A deeply jarring statistic of the flu pandemic was that over 30% of the deaths occurred in India which lost six percent of its population. Compare that with the COVID-19 pandemic which affected over 43 million people and officially claimed over 700,000 lives as of October 1, 2021. Even discounting for a politically expedient undercount of the dead and pegging the number at what experts put at the more realistic figure in the range of three million or so, it is still much better than the flu pandemic.

There has been some debate over whether democracies such as the United States and India handle massive public health crises better or totalitarian systems such as China and Russia. The answer as shown by the COVID-19 pandemic is complex. Both India and the United States went through a period of disastrous mishandling during the early phase of the pandemic in 2020 while China, in whose city of Wuhan in the central Chinese province of Hubei the virus originated, managed to control it via some draconian restrictions on people's movement as well as transmission of any worthwhile news or data to the outside world. If an alien civilization were monitoring the pandemic, they may be misled to think that the pandemic began either in India or America given the utter chaos triggered in both countries.

In this context, the figures from China as quoted by Johns Hopkins University's tracker are both intriguing and mystifying. According to the World Health Organization (WHO)'s dashboard, in China, from January 3, 2020, to 1 October 2021, there have been 124,673 confirmed cases of COVID-19 with 5,691 deaths. That is an extraordinary example of state control if true. If the country where the virus originated accounts for barely 0.05 percent of the total global cases and a little over 0.1 percent of the global deaths, it can broadly mean two things. One is that China has been exceptionally efficient and successful in controlling the spread of the virus within its own border even as it jumped to the rest of the world and devastated economies and peoples. The other is that the figures are profoundly manipulated to the extent of being just pure lies. Since the WHO and even the Johns Hopkins tracker accept the figures at their face value it is hard to refute them in the absence of direct, on-the-ground access to the realities there. Incidentally, the Johns Hopkins tracker puts the figures even lower for China at 108,495 cases and 4,849 deaths since the pandemic started.

One extraordinary success story in the aftermath of the pandemic has been the total number of vaccine doses administered by October 1, 2021. The number was more than 6.2 billion with China alone claiming over 2.2 billion doses for over 74 percent of its population or over one billion people. India, regarded as the world's vaccine central and pharmaceutical hub, had after the initial disaster managed to administer 870 million doses. The United States was the third-highest in administering doses of over 380 million.

Although India had begun to turn the tide around by October 2021, its prime minister Narendra Modi and his administration too ran into its most serious existential crisis for the better part of 2020 as it piled ineptitude on top ineptitude while dealing with the crisis. In a country where the public health infrastructure has long been woefully ramshackle and inadequate; it was not long before the ravages of the pandemic became evident quickly. For weeks and months, the Indian media reported breathlessly about a mortal shortage of oxygen. Images of people dying by the roadsides, in ambulances, at homes, and all manners of public places for want of oxygen were all over the broadcast and print media. The macabre dance of death was topped by the images of bodies floating in the Ganga River in the state of Uttar Pradesh. This was disturbingly reminiscent of the poet Nirala's observations about the influenza pandemic of 1918–1919.

Many reasons were given for families leaving their dead relatives floating either in the river or on the banks, including poverty preventing them from being able to cremate. Many were barely buried on the banks of the Ganga.

This complete collapse at various levels of governance exposed the Modi government to unprecedented opprobrium with even some of the prime minister's most ardent supporters offering a semblance of criticism. Unlike in America, a fellow democracy, in India the politicization over the pandemic was not necessarily about whether the pandemic was real but a lack of access to hospital beds, oxygen cylinders, inadequate ambulances, and so on. Given the country's millennial sense of fatalism among its people, there was a large number of Indians, especially in rural India that did not wear masks throughout the pandemic.

Considering this all-around failure not just to anticipate contingencies by the Modi government but even poor public health infrastructure, officially India appeared to have been spared the scale of death and destruction that should have happened. According to the Johns Hopkins tracker, as of October 5, 2021, India had reported a total of over 33 million cases and nearly 450,000 deaths. Unofficially and according to many respected global experts, there was a serious underreporting of the numbers for politically expedient reasons and those who died could easily be five to eight times the actual figure.

Apart from the pandemic's many obvious fallouts in terms of its impact on governance, public health policy, politics, culture, and economy, one particularly interesting aspect of the crisis has been the role that the global media played in both reporting it from many different angles but even exposing some glaring shortcomings in the way China, where it originated, mishandled it and the World Health Organization (WHO) went along with early Chinese assertions without much pushback.

Before we get into how the pandemic has upended the world, it is important to get a glimpse of how its overall economic impact will be.

According to the World Economic Situation and Prospects (WESP), mid-2021 report of the United Nations, "While the global growth outlook has improved, led by robust rebound in China and the United States, surging COVID-19 infections and inadequate vaccination progress in many countries threaten a broad-based recovery of the world economy."

The year 2020 saw a sharp contraction of 3.6 percent in the global economy but it was projected to expand by 5.4 percent in 2021.

"Amid rapid vaccinations and continued fiscal and monetary support measures, China and the United States—the two largest economies— are on the path to recovery," the WESP report said.

"In contrast, the growth outlook in several countries in South Asia, sub-Saharan Africa, and Latin America and the Caribbean, remains fragile and uncertain. For many countries, economic output is only projected to return to pre-pandemic levels in 2022 or 2023," it said.

That part is the worrisome one because together those countries account for a total of over three billion people (1.3 billion in India, 1.14 billion in sub-Saharan Africa, and nearly 670 million in Latin America and the Caribbean.) Any prolongation in their return to pre-pandemic levels could be problematic for the global economy.

The WESP quoted UN Chief Economist Elliott Harris as saying, "Vaccine inequity between countries and regions is posing a significant risk to an already uneven and fragile global recovery.

Timely and universal access to COVID-19 vaccinations will mean the difference between ending the pandemic promptly and placing the world economy on the trajectory of a resilient recovery, or losing many more years of growth, development and opportunities."

On the global trade front, the news was encouraging, according to the WESP. "Global merchandise trade has already surpassed pre-pandemic levels, buoyed by strong demand for electrical and electronic equipment, personal protective equipment, and other manufactured goods.

"Manufacturing-dependent economies have fared better, both during the crisis and the recovery period, but a quick rebound looks unlikely for tourism- and commodity-dependent economies, the report underscored.

"Trade-in services, in particular tourism, will remain depressed amid slow lifting of restrictions on international travel and fear of new waves of infection in many developing countries." However, perhaps the most worrisome aspect of the report was that women were the worst hit by the pandemic despite being at the forefront of the fight against the pandemic.

The U.N. said women have also been hit the hardest in a number of ways, including bearing the brunt of unpaid domestic and care work. "They remain underrepresented in pandemic-related decision-making and in economic policy responses to the crisis. While the pandemic has reduced labor force participation by 2 per cent worldwide, compared to only 0.2 per cent during the global financial crisis of 2007–2008, more women than men were forced to leave the work force altogether, further widening gender gaps in employment and wages, the report highlighted," it said.

"The pandemic has pushed nearly 58 million women and girls into extreme poverty, dealing a huge blow to poverty reduction efforts worldwide, and exacerbated gender gaps in income, wealth and education, impeding progress on gender equality," said Hamid Rashid, the Chief of the Global Economic Monitoring Branch at the UN Department of Economic and Social Affairs, and the lead author of the report.

"Fiscal and monetary measures to steer recovery must take into account the differentiated impact of the crisis on different population groups, including women, to ensure an economic recovery that is inclusive and resilient," he added.

Over two years after the pandemic, the global output was projected to be slashed by $8.5 trillion, according to the WESP, "Wiping out nearly all gains of the previous four years."

It may seem intuitive that the pandemic would have pushed large numbers of people across the world into extreme poverty. In January 2021 as experts began to look back at 2020 to assess the number of people pushed into extreme poverty, the World Bank's Global Economic Prospect (GEP) initially estimated that between 119 and 124 million people could slide into extreme poverty. However, the GEP was revised in June 2021 to peg the number at 97 million, which represented a reduction of about 20 million people.

The bank said, "In 2021, we project global poverty to decrease by about 21 million people compared with 2020. This represents exactly the same decline we had expected would occur in 2021 before the pandemic hit. The implications of this estimate are that global poverty is projected to decline, and the pace of reduction is returning to the pre-pandemic trend. In that sense, one could say that global poverty may be turning the corner on the pandemic in 2021. Still, this does not mean that we are getting back to the level of poverty we had anticipated in 2021 before the pandemic spread. In fact, because the pace of reduction is similar to what we expected before the pandemic spread, the recovery taking place will not be sufficient to close the gap the pandemic is estimated to have caused in 2020."

"Globally, the increase in poverty that occurred in 2020 due to COVID still lingers, and the COVID-induced poor in 2021 continues to be 97 million people," the bank added.

And then in a twist typical of such complex assessments, the bank said this, "If global poverty continues to reduce at the pace we expected before the pandemic, every year there will be tens of millions of people living in poverty because of the initial fallout from the pandemic."

In that assessment, the bank offered this as one of the explanations for this seeming dichotomy, "When the pandemic broke out, many developing countries responded in ways similar to high-income countries; by locking down major parts of their economy. These lockdowns decreased incomes and employment, causing an increase in extreme poverty. In 2021, the appetite for lockdowns has been smaller. This may have limited the economic consequences at the cost of increased COVID cases and COVID-related deaths. This pattern is reflected in the OxCGRT stringency index, which captures countries' response to the pandemic including school and work closure, travel bans, partial or full lockdowns. In May 2020, on average 25 out of 27 low-income countries in OxCGRT had a stringency index value higher than 50, whereas in May 2021, on average 10 low-income countries crossed that threshold. In addition, the pandemic is receding in many high-income countries, and economic activity is once again on the rise. This could lower poverty in low- and middle-income countries if the rise in economic activity spurs demand for their products and commodities."

Notwithstanding this, it is clear that COVID has led to the first rise in extreme poverty in a generation as pointed out by the United Nations statistics. A summary accompanying a UN report said, "The effects of the coronavirus disease 2019 (COVID-19) pandemic have reversed much of the progress made in reducing poverty, with global extreme poverty rising in 2020 for the first time since the Asian financial crisis of the late 1990s. Even before COVID-19, the world was not on track to achieve the goal of ending poverty by 2030, and without immediate and significant action, it will remain beyond reach. The crisis has demonstrated more clearly than ever the importance of disaster preparedness and robust social protection systems. While the number of countries with disaster risk reduction strategies has increased substantially, and many temporary social protection measures have been put in place in response to the pandemic, increased efforts are needed on both fronts to ensure the most vulnerable are protected."

The UN said, "Before the COVID-19 pandemic, the share of the world's population living in extreme poverty fell from 10.1 per cent in 2015 to 9.3 per cent in 2017. This means that the number of people living on less than $1.90 per day dropped from 741 million to 689 million. However, the rate of reduction had slowed to less than half a percentage point annually between 2015 and 2017, compared with one percentage point annually between 1990 and 2015.

"The pandemic has compounded the threats to progress raised by conflict and climate change. Estimates suggest that 2020 saw an increase of between 119 million and 124 million global poor, of whom 60 per cent are in Southern Asia. Now casts point to the first rise in the extreme poverty rate since 1998, from 8.4 per cent in 2019 to 9.5 per cent in 2020, undoing the progress made since 2016. The impacts of the pandemic will not be short-lived. Based on current projections, the global poverty rate is expected to be 7 per cent [around 600 million people] in 2030, missing the target of eradicating poverty."

Bare statistics may not immediately tell us the staggering number of those living in abject poverty but as a single entity. If all the 600 million poor people living in poverty were in a single country, they would form the world's third most populous nation. Living on less than $1.90 a day is a figure that would be incomprehensible for people in North America and across Europe but that is a daily reality for some 600 million-plus people.

Taken together the pandemic has seriously upended global models of governance both in democracies as well as totalitarian states. What is going to profoundly compound this is the looming consequences of climate change.

Even though a detailed discussion on the effects of climate change is beyond the scope of this book in so much as it dovetails into crises such as the COVID-19 pandemic and how it upends governance models it is important to cite some of the observations of the Intergovernmental Panel on Climate Change (IPCC) contained in its sixth report. They are as follows:

- It is unequivocal that human influence has warmed the atmosphere, ocean, and land. Widespread and rapid changes in the atmosphere, ocean, cryosphere, and biosphere have occurred.

- The scale of recent changes across the climate system as a whole and the present state of many aspects of the climate system are unprecedented over many centuries to many thousands of years.

- Human-induced climate change is already affecting many weather and climate extremes in every region across the globe. Evidence of observed changes in extremes such as heatwaves, heavy precipitation, droughts, and tropical cyclones, and in particular, their attribution to human influence has strengthened since the Fifth Assessment Report (AR5).

- Improved knowledge of climate processes, paleoclimate evidence, and the response of the climate system to increasing radiative forcing gives the best estimate of equilibrium climate sensitivity of 3°C.

The IPCC report draws up possible climate futures as follows:

- Global surface temperature will continue to increase until at least the mid-century under all emissions scenarios considered. Global warming of 1.5°C and 2°C will be exceeded during the 21st century unless deep reductions in carbon dioxide (CO_2) and other greenhouse gas emissions occur in the coming decades.

- Many changes in the climate system become larger in direct relation to increasing global warming. They include increases in the frequency and intensity of hot extremes, marine heatwaves, and heavy precipitation, agricultural and ecological droughts in some regions, and proportion of intense tropical cyclones, as well as reductions in Arctic Sea ice, snow cover, and permafrost.

- Continued global warming is projected to further intensify the global water cycle, including its variability, global monsoon precipitation, and the severity of wet and dry events.

- Under scenarios with increasing CO_2 emissions, the ocean and land carbon sinks are projected to be less effective at slowing the accumulation of CO_2 in the atmosphere. B.5 many changes due to past and future greenhouse gas emissions are irreversible for centuries to millennia, especially changes in the ocean, ice sheets, and global sea level.

With global pressures mounting on so many fronts, be it waves of pandemics and epidemics or a wide variety of consequences of climate change such as massive storms, raging forest fires, extensive flooding, intense droughts, debilitated heat and cold waves, and rising sea levels, everything has a direct bearing on the way ideas about leadership have to be fundamentally overhauled. The fact that the world's two giant democracies, America and India experienced comparable COVID-related failures—from the shortage of hospital beds to the shortage of oxygen, for instance—shows leaders across the world will have to retool themselves in order to meet a whole new set of challenges of the twenty-first century. Since relatively short-duration crises such as those resulting from a pandemic or the much longer-term existential threats from climate change operate well outside the realm of ideological divides, prejudices, and predilections responding to them from the standpoint of the politics of the nineteenth and twentieth centuries will simply not work.

There is now a desperate need for the world to come together to develop some globally uniform standards of what constitutes good governance because increasingly we will experience problems which defy boundaries and operate well outside the outdated ideas of nation-states. In that context, perhaps the United Nations needs to rethink its role and start a serious movement to help engender global standards of good governance and that should become a regular feature of the annual United Nations General Assembly in New York. Unless the world acts in concert, often as a single entity, the twenty-first century has the potential to permanently upend the progress achieved in the two rounds of the industrial revolution since 1760 when it began in Britain.

Take for instance this particular passage from a United Nations report by the Statistics Division of its Department of Economic and Social Affairs, "Social protection measures are fundamental to preventing and reducing poverty across the life cycle. Nevertheless, by 2020, only 46.9 per cent of the global population were effectively covered by at least one social protection cash benefit, leaving as many as 4 billion people without a social safety net. The COVID-19 crisis has demonstrated the importance of social protection systems to protect people's health, jobs and incomes, as well as the consequences of high coverage gaps. As a result, many new social protection measures were introduced in 2020: between 1 February and 31 December, the governments of 209 countries and territories announced more than 1,600 such measures in response to the crisis, but almost all (94.7 per cent) were short term in nature.

"Before the pandemic, most of the population (85.4 per cent) in high-income countries was effectively covered by at least one social protection benefit, compared with just over one tenth (13.4 per cent) in low-income countries. The coverage gap is even greater for those considered vulnerable, only 7.8 per cent of whom were covered by social assistance in low-income countries."

Social protection, so uneven across the world as it is, is expected to come under an even greater strain as the world battles so many diverse crises and fails to meet them for the largest number of people. Unlike perhaps any other time in history, the twenty-first century is fraught with both serious challenges and enormous possibilities for leaders across the world to invent a whole new model or governance and a whole new idiom of communicating it.

What compounded the global situation by the last week of November 2021 was the rise of yet another mutation out of South Africa called omicron. Early reports suggested that omicron was unusual in that it had 50 mutations, 32 of which were on the spike protein, a club-shaped structure that helps it attach to human cells.

A couple of days after its discovery, the World Health Organization (WHO) said this about omicron's transmissibility and the severity of the disease it caused.

Transmissibility: *"It is not yet clear whether omicron is more transmissible (e.g., more easily spread from person to person) compared to other variants, including delta. The number of people testing positive has risen in areas of South Africa affected by this variant, but epidemiologic studies are underway to understand if it is because of omicron or other factors."*

Severity of disease: "It is not yet clear whether infection with omicron causes more severe disease compared to infections with other variants, including delta. Preliminary data suggests that there are increasing rates of hospitalization in South Africa, but this may be due to increasing overall numbers of people becoming infected, rather than a result of specific infection with omicron. There is currently no information to suggest that symptoms associated with omicron are different from those from other variants. Initial reported infections were among university students—younger individuals who tend to have more mild disease—but understanding the level of severity of the omicron variant will take days to several weeks. All variants of COVID-19, including the delta variant that is dominant worldwide, can cause severe disease or death, in particular for the most vulnerable people, and thus prevention is always key."

It had become clear by the end of 2021 that this COVID-19 will become diffused but never quite go away, acquiring a more endemic nature like other viruses. In the process though it will leave the world order significantly disrupted.

References

(Editor's note: This chapter is exempt from APA7 referencing style)

- https://www.bc.edu/bc-web/bcnews/science-tech-and-health/biology-and-genetics/tracking-ancient-viruses1.html (How long viruses have existed?)

- https://news.un.org/en/story/2021/09/1098942 (The rise of the Mu variant)

- https://www.politico.com/news/2021/04/23/trump-bleach-one-year-484399 (President Trump advocating by implication the use of bleach etc.)

- https://www.usatoday.com/story/news/health/2021/09/22/covid-vaccines-mandates-cases-deaths-biden-administration/5805943001/ (Deaths in the new wave)

- https://www.nytimes.com/2021/10/01/us/us-covid-deaths-700k.html (Spike in 2021 deaths)

- https://www.cdc.gov/flu/pandemic-resources/1918-commemoration/1918-pandemic-history.htm (Background about the 1918 flu)

- https://www.bbc.com/news/world-asia-india-51904019 (Background about 1918 flu)

- https://www.un.org/development/desa/dpad/wp-content/uploads/sites/45/publication/WESP_MID_2021_PR_E.pdf (Global economic projection)

- https://www.un.org/en/desa/covid-19-slash-global-economic-output-85-trillion-over-next-two-years (Global economic projection)

- https://blogs.worldbank.org/opendata/updated-estimates-impact-covid-19-global-poverty-turning-corner-pandemic-2021 (The pandemic's impact on global poverty)

- https://unstats.un.org/sdgs/report/2021/goal-01/ (UN statistics on global poverty)

INDEX

A

adaptive capacity, 19–21, 26, 28, 30

Akpan, I., 181

algorithms, 274, 277, 286, 289, 292, 294

Al Kahtani, M., 286

alpha coronaviruses, 250

Alpha variant, 45–46

America, xli, 308, 310, 313, 315, 323

Anderies, J. M., 17

Aristotle, 205

AstraZeneca, 44, 47, 263, 267, 276

Axelrod, R., 28–29

B

Baccini, L., 126

BCG (Boston Consulting Group), 97, 105, 260

Bender, A., 13–14

beta coronaviruses, 250, 257

Bhattacharyya, D. K., 285–86

Brazil, 103–4, 113

Brem, A., 172–74

Broduer, A., 126

businesses
    small, 126–27, 202, 214
    traditional, 87, 96

C

Canada, 100, 103, 113

CARES Act (Coronavirus Aid, Relief and Economic Security Act), 43, 112, 126, 231

Catastrophic Collapse, 4, 31

CCM (critical care medicine), 222–23, 241

CDC (Center for Disease Control), xliii–xliv, 40–42, 45, 47–48, 66, 139, 225, 235, 239, 252, 257–58, 263, 265, 268, 311

CEPI (Coalition for Epidemic Preparedness Innovations), 267

CFR (case fatality rates), 59

challenges, xxxvi, 29, 39, 98, 144, 149–50, 163, 168, 170, 193, 195, 197, 241, 264, 273, 276, 281, 283, 323

change management, xlv, li, 195, 197–98, 202, 273–74, 276–77, 279–81, 283, 286–87, 291, 297

chest CT scan, 252

China, 3, 40–41, 43, 122, 161, 224–25, 236, 248–49, 255, 278, 313–14, 316

citizens, 57, 122–23, 126–27, 130, 138, 193–94, 198–203, 206–9, 211–12, 215–16, 218, 227, 308

climate change, 10–12, 14, 20, 22, 24, 212, 321, 323

complexity, xli, xlvi, xlix–li, 1–3, 5, 20, 22, 70, 193–94, 200, 204, 214, 282–83, 285

coronavirus, xxxix, xlii–xliii, 40, 90, 111, 145, 197, 211, 248–52, 254–55, 271

countries

developing, 25, 97, 267, 317, 319

high-income, 319, 324

low-income, 319, 324

COVID-19, *xxxix–xlii, xlvii–l, 29, 40–43, 47–58, 62, 84–86, 90–92, 95–102, 109–114, 122, 129–133, 136–139, 144–146, 150–162, 168, 170–184, 193–202, 210–218, 222, 226–236, 241, 248–259, 268, 276, 285, 305–307, 313, 320, 325*

vaccine, 43, 236, 238, 258–61, 266–68

variants, 234, 258–59, 262, 269, 325

D

decision-making, 14, 16, 18, 21–22, 26, 200

Deimler, M., 20–21

Deliverloo, 109

Delta variant, 46, 216, 234–35, 257, 310, 325

DNA (deoxyribonucleic acid), 293

computers, 294, 296

computing, 293–94

E

Eastin, J., 25

economic losses, 139

EIDL (Economic Injury Disaster Loan), 112

Engle, N. L., 19–20

entrepreneurs, xxvi, 148, 177, 179, 181–82

entrepreneurship, 148, 170–71, 179–81, 183–84

envelope proteins, 254

essential workers, 130, 227

F

FDA (Food and Drug Administration), 47, 262–63

fear, 72, 124–25, 134, 138–39, 193, 196, 201, 297

Fiksel, J., 14

Folke, C., 8

freelancers, 86, 94–95, 112

freelancing, 86–87, 94–95

G

game theory, xxvi, 27–29

GCR (Gauteng City-Region), 16

GDP (gross domestic product), 135

GEP (Global Economic Prospect), 318

Gershenson, C., 12–13

GFC (global financial crisis), 24, 123, 317

GGSP (Gauteng Green Strategic Programme), 16

gig economy, 84–89, 91–93, 95–100, 102–11, 114–15

gig workers, 85–86, 88–89, 92–94, 99–100, 106–7, 110–11, 113, 115

Gill, R., 283

global events, unexpected, 38–39, 61, 67

global health systems, xliv, 305

golden ratio, 274

Götz, G., 16

growth, 26, 95–96, 104–5, 110, 149, 151, 170, 178, 180–81, 284, 317

GSO (guided self-organization), 10–13

H

Hall, T. J., 15

Hayes, J., 285

HCWs (healthcare workers), 199, 210, 222–29, 231, 234, 237–40

female, 228

healthcare sector, 229, 231, 295

Hilbert space, 289

Hoek, R. V., 285

I

IFR (infection fatality rates), 59

immune response, 260–62, 268, 275

Impact of COVID-19, *86, 90, 91, 92, 93, 95, 105–107, 113, 144, 151, 161, 170, 180, 213*

India, 1, 3, 45–46, 105–6, 114, 144–45, 149–52, 156–59, 161–63, 168, 170–71, 175, 177–78, 182–84, 235, 257, 267, 307, 311, 313–16, 323

Indians, 161, 171, 184, 315

influenza pandemic, 305, 310, 315

J

Johns Hopkins tracker, 314–15

Johnson & Johnson, 46–47, 262–63, 273, 276

K

Kuckertz, A., 148, 180–81

L

Lauer, T., 283

leadership, 19, 39, 195, 198, 201, 203, 217–18, 283, 323

Lemos, M. C., 8, 21

Lewin, K., 217, 284

Lifton, R., 196

lockdowns, 41, 48, 58, 123, 125, 197, 200, 202, 211–12, 214, 216, 319

LTG (Limits to Growth), 24–25

M

McEvoy, D., 22

medical community, 248–49, 252, 268

membrane proteins, 40, 254

MERS (Middle East respiratory syndrome), xliv, 249–50

Michael & Susan Dell Foundation, 97

Moderna, 44, 46–47, 235, 262, 265–67, 273, 276

Mrotzek, M., 23

Munang, R., 8

mutations, xli, 45, 196, 209, 216, 234, 256, 269, 307, 325

N

NE (Nash equilibria), 28–30

Nelson, D. R., 19

new normal, xxxvi, 38–39, 60–61, 73, 90, 122, 137, 140, 150, 158, 171, 176, 184, 241, 280

New Normal, 171

NIH (National Institutes of Health), 43, 45, 250, 257

Novavax vaccine, 263–64

O

OECD (Organization for Economic Co-operation and Development), 87, 96, 111–12

omicron, xl, 45–46, 234, 325

organizational change, 209, 285–86

organizational collapse, 24

Ossimitz, G., 23

OWS (Operation Warp Speed), 43, 275

Oxford-AstraZeneca vaccine, 263, 265

P

pandemic, xxxv–xxxvi, xxxix–xliv, xlvi–xlvii, 38–39, 41–43, 48–50, 55–57, 60–61, 74–75, 84–87, 90–92, 95–104, 106, 109–11, 113–16, 121–36, 144–45, 149–51, 168–73, 182–84, 193–94, 198–204, 208–10, 213–16, 222–23, 226–35, 273–76, 279–97, 308–10, 313–21

flu, 310–13

global, 42, 121–22, 134, 137–38, 144–45, 148, 171

PCR (Polymerase chain reaction), xlii–xliii, 51, 55, 249, 252–53, 272

PD (prisoner's dilemma), 27

Pfizer, 44, 46–47, 264, 267, 273, 276, 281

Pfizer-BioNTech vaccine, 262

PGGs (public goods games), 29–30

policy measures, 150, 168

polyploidy, 256–57, 272

poverty, 319–21

  extreme, 200, 318–20

  global, 318–19

PPE (personal protection equipment), 116, 127, 130, 160, 199, 215, 225–26, 231–32, 234

Q

QCC (quantum computational chemistry), 290

quantum computer development, 279, 284, 286, 297

quantum computers, 273–87, 290–94, 296–97

quantum computing, 276–77, 280, 282, 285–86, 292, 294, 297

R

Ram, I. G., 217

Ram, K., 213

RBNs (random Boolean networks), 12

Reeves, M., 20–21

resilience, 7, 9, 14, 17, 19, 22, 177

  entrepreneurial, 177

resilience framework, 9–10, 19, 24

resilience management, 8

resistance to change, 208–9, 282, 284, 296

resources, 2, 10, 130, 193–94, 199–200, 202, 207, 233, 242, 267, 281, 283

retroviruses, 306–7

RNA (ribonucleic acid), 262, 272

robustness, 10, 13, 19, 21

Rogers, T., 229

RRSA (resilience, robustness, sustainability, and adaptive-capacity) model, xxvi, 6, 23

RT (Respiratory therapists), 236

S

SARS (severe acute respiratory syndrome), xliv, 42, 224–25, 249–50

Schäffler, A., 16

SESs (socio-ecological systems), 7–8, 23

shutdowns, 58, 115, 123, 126, 131–32, 138–39

SIG (SARS-CoV-2 Interagency Group), 45

Slaper, T. F., 15

social distancing, 129, 136–37, 207

South Africa, xxvi, xli, 46, 197, 211–12, 267, 325

spike proteins, 254, 262–64, 271, 325

Start-up India, 168–69

startups, 156, 279

stock market, 133, 135, 137

superposition, 294

supply chains, 70–73, 76, 177, 296, 305

sustainability, 14, 16, 18, 71, 175

sustainability management, 18

sustainable technology, 17

T

TBL (triple-bottom-line), 15–16

technology entrepreneurship, l, 144–45, 148–51, 157–59, 163, 170–72, 175, 178–80, 183–84

technology start-ups, l, 144–45, 149–51, 156–59, 161, 163–64, 168–71, 175–76, 178, 180–81, 183–84

Turner, G. M., 24–25

U

UK (United Kingdom), 47, 86, 91, 98, 107–11, 114–15, 212, 263

unemployment, 127–29, 134–35, 137

rates, 122, 128–29, 131

US (United States), 5, 41, 44, 52–54, 56, 58, 60, 64, 86–87, 94–95, 98, 112, 121–22, 126–27, 131, 139, 149, 225, 233, 237, 257, 266, 268, 307, 310, 313–14, 316

V

vaccinations, 49, 138–39, 162, 226, 240, 263

vaccines

mRNA, 233, 262

protein subunit, 261

viral vector, 260–61, 263

Verschuur, J., 61–62

viral gene sequencing, 253

VOC (Variant of Concern), xl, 45–46

W

Wang, D., 61

WESP (World Economic Situation and Prospects), 316–18

WFH (work from home), 62–65, 74–75, 87, 90, 216–17, 227

Whitacre, J., 13–14

WHO (World Health Organization), xl, xliv, 40, 43, 45, 122, 199–200, 307, 313, 316, 325

Wuhan, China, 40–41, 122, 196–97, 214, 225, 248

www.ingramcontent.com/pod-product-compliance
Lightning Source LLC
Chambersburg PA
CBHW021348210526
45463CB00001B/19